THE

LOST BOOK OF NATIVE AMERICAN HERBALIST'S BIBLE

The Ultimate Collection of Herbs Loose Leaves and Remedies for Common Ailments

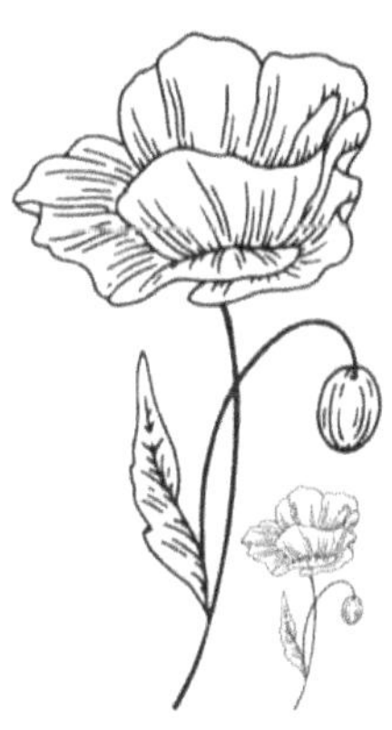

Sage Herbal

Limitation of Liability/Disclaimer of Warranty:

The publisher and the author provide no guarantees regarding the accuracy or completeness of the contents of this work. They specifically disclaim all warranties, including those related to fitness for a specific purpose. There are no warranties that can be created or extended through sales or promotional materials. Please note that the advice and strategies provided may not be suitable for all situations. This work is sold with the understanding that the publisher is not providing medical, legal, or other professional advice or services. If you need professional assistance, it is advisable to seek the services of a competent professional person. The publisher and author are not responsible for any damages that may occur. Please note that the inclusion of an individual, organization, or website as a citation or potential source of further information in this work does not imply endorsement by the author or publisher. The information or recommendations provided by these sources are not necessarily endorsed. Additionally, it is important for readers to note that any websites mentioned in this work may have undergone changes or become unavailable since the time of writing.

ISBN: 979-8-8693-6161-5

Author: Sage Herbal

Book Title: The Lost Book of Native American Herbalist's Bible: The Ultimate Collection of Herbs Loose Leaves and Remedies for Common Ailments

Introduction

Herbal medicine has a rich and ancient history that predates modern pharmaceuticals by thousands of years.

It is a significant aspect of alternative medicine, and proves beneficial in preventing and treating various common ailments.

The natural world is abundant with a wide variety of herbs that have remarkable healing properties. With guidance and knowledge, anyone can harness the power of herbs to alleviate discomfort and support the healing process.

As a child in the mountains of Montana, I was captivated by the tales of Native Americans who possessed incredible healing knowledge. They would harness the power of the wild plants that thrived near our home to create remedies for various ailments. It wasn't until I reached adulthood that I started to explore teas beyond the basic peppermint and chamomile varieties. Today, I take great pleasure in cultivating a wide variety of aromatic herbs in my garden and the lush hardwood forest that surrounds my home. I thoroughly enjoy strolling through the woods and along riverbanks, admiring the medicinal plants and appreciating their beauty and effectiveness as I breathe in their delightful fragrances. Whenever I'm not feeling my best, I can usually rely on the plants I've harvested and prepared to take care of myself.

Certain herbal remedies utilize plant parts in their fresh, natural state. Some prefer store-bought extracts, while others enjoy making their own compounds at home. Through careful research and consideration, I have taken control of my own health and effectively addressed minor ailments before they escalate and necessitate medical attention. Now you can also experience it.

Buying medicinal herbs has become incredibly convenient, with popular options readily available at pharmacies and big-box stores. Health food stores provide a wide range of whole herbs, as well as tinctures, teas, ointments, and other products that offer an alternative to pharmaceuticals.

It may be unexpected to discover that many traditional pharmaceuticals have their origins in herbal medicine.

Aspirin is derived from willow bark, while morphine is meticulously extracted from opium poppies. Quinine, an essential medication for treating malaria, is derived from the bark of the cinchona tree. Digoxin, a powerful drug used in cardiac cases, is sourced from the stunning yet toxic foxglove plant. Several pharmaceuticals are derived from plants or synthesized using compounds that closely resemble natural substances.

However, mainstream medicine tends to favor synthetic drugs due to their standardized formulations, purity, and convenience. It's no surprise that prescription pharmaceuticals have gained a highly sought-after reputation. This book does not aim to diminish their significance. Nevertheless, it is crucial to bear in mind that in the United States, herbs are classified as dietary supplements and are subject to corresponding regulations when sold commercially. Thus, when opting for a natural approach to treating an ailment, there is no need to acquire a prescription, unlike synthetic drugs. Instead, you can utilize a herbal poultice, apply a basic cream or oil, or consume a tincture or tea.

Although herbs are potent, they typically lack the long-lasting side effects commonly associated with pharmaceuticals. They enhance the body's natural healing process; especially when combined with rest, they improve our recovery ability. Several herbs can enhance the immune system, facilitating the body's utilization of its innate defenses to combat viruses and infections.

Compiling a comprehensive inventory of medicinal plants would require a monumental endeavor, and even then, it would be exceedingly challenging to encompass the full range of properties exhibited by each individual plant. With a wide array of options to choose from, it can be challenging to determine which herbs to use, despite the abundance of detailed guides available.

This book stands out from the rest. Here, you'll discover a comprehensive guide to utilizing widely recognized and potent medicinal herbs. You can easily find all of them online or at your local health food store. It's highly probable that you can discover some of them flourishing just a stone's throw away from your doorstep. There might be a few hiding in your spice cabinet! Whether you are new to the world of herbal medicine or have already started to experience the therapeutic benefits of plants, you'll find this book to be valuable.

Chapter I

Herbal Medicine in History

In the past, people relied on natural remedies to address their health issues, long before pharmaceutical companies came into existence. Whether this was a natural progression or one found through experimentation, herbal medicine is not a recent development. What is noteworthy is its comeback, particularly in light of widely reported issues with mainstream medications. However, let's start from the very beginning. Throughout history, diverse cultures have harnessed the power of their local flora to create plant-based remedies. Each continent's rich ecosystem has provided a wealth of unique remedies, tailored to the specific needs of different countries. Even in this day and age, advanced medical treatments and medications remain out of reach for many people in various parts of the world. As a result, herbal healers continue to play a vital role in public health.

Africa

Medical texts have been around for thousands of years. The ancient Egyptian works known as the Edwin Smith Papyrus and Papyrus Ebers, named after their discoverers, contain detailed descriptions of anatomy, records of injuries, and knowledge of herbal pharmacology. They also include designs for medical and surgical instruments.

African traditional medicine values the use of herbal remedies, drawing from a rich natural pharmacy of around 4,000 native plants. Pharmaceutical companies have come to appreciate the value of Africa's herbal medicines. They are now collaborating with local practitioners and studying traditional remedies to discover bioactive agents that can be utilized in the development of modern synthetic medicines.

Asia

Early literature documenting the utilization of Chinese herbs was discovered in Changsha, China, within the Mawangdui Han tombs that were sealed in 168 BCE. Known as Wushi'er Bingfang, or Recipes for 52 Ailments, this comprehensive list of prescriptions offers more than 250 remedies for a wide range of ailments, including hemorrhoids and warts.

Traditional Asian medicine encompasses a range of practices such as massage, exercise, acupuncture, herbal treatments, and dietary therapy. These practices were standardized in China during the 1950s but have a long history, dating back to about 1100 BCE, when numerous herbal remedies were described.

By the end of the sixteenth century, traditional Asian physicians had around 1,900 remedies available to them. Fast forward to the end of the twentieth century, and the Chinese materia medica had expanded to include a staggering 12,800 different drugs.

In India, a significant sourcebook known as the Atharva Veda established the principles of Ayurveda, a healing practice that originated around 1200 BCE. This system is still being utilized in the present day.

Ancient Middle Eastern physicians were knowledgeable herbalists who shared their wisdom with Greek and Persian scholars. Eventually, Arabs generously shared their knowledge with European crusaders, who then returned to their own countries with this valuable information.

Australia

European ships first arrived in Australia in the 1600s, but it was in 1788 that a collision occurred between indigenous and imperialist cultures when Britain's First Fleet brought around 1,500 people to Sydney. In the past, indigenous communities heavily relied on herbal medicine.

Nevertheless, due to their cultural reliance on oral history, which involves storytelling, singing, and dancing rituals, there are no written records available regarding Australia's earliest herbal medicines. With the passing of the last practicing elders, the number of rituals dwindles and valuable knowledge about the continent's medicinal flora is being lost.

Today, indigenous aboriginal medicine is commonly known as bush medicine. The practice focuses on traditional treatments that make use of Australian leaves and seeds. Local treatments like native grapes and banksia flowers are highly regarded, while eucalyptus and turmeric have gained global recognition for their value.

Europe

Early Greek and Roman physicians were highly respected for their extensive knowledge of herbs. A significant amount of their knowledge had been inherited from Egyptian physicians. Regarded as a pioneer in the field of medicine, Hippocrates received his education from esteemed Egyptian priest-doctors. After the decline of the Roman Empire, scientific advancements came to a standstill, resulting in a significant loss of knowledge in the field of herbal medicine. With the rise in trade with other civilizations, there was a renewed interest in the study of medicinal herbs. During the Renaissance, European nobles made extensive efforts to collect and organize a wealth of knowledge in their libraries. Additionally, they dedicated themselves to gathering the most valuable botanical specimens in their gardens. In the sixteenth and seventeenth centuries, universities offered courses on herbalism and botany, where they established "physic" gardens to cultivate medicinal plants.

In 1652, Nicholas Culpeper released The English Physician, a comprehensive catalog of herbal remedies found in England. The book was designed to cater to a wide audience, focusing on the use of herbs to treat everyday ailments rather than relying on costly remedies prescribed by medical professionals.

With the advent of the scientific age, herbal remedies lost their popularity. Herbal remedies have experienced a resurgence in popularity throughout Europe, despite being overshadowed by modern drugs for a period of time.

North America

For countless generations, Native American and First Nations communities have embraced the power of natural remedies, prioritizing holistic well-being by nurturing the body, rejuvenating the spirit, and achieving mental harmony. According to ancient oral traditions, the earliest healers acquired their knowledge of medicinal herbs by closely observing sick animals. Due to the lack of written records, it is difficult to determine how native North Americans utilized herbs prior to their initial interaction with Europeans. The information was primarily transmitted through oral tradition. However, the situation shifted when indigenous people generously shared their natural remedies with the new settlers, who happened to possess knowledge of European herbal medicine. Indeed, numerous colonists brought their cherished healing plants along as they journeyed to the New World. Several of these plants have become established throughout North America and can be found growing alongside the continent's native flora. Over time, herbal remedies gradually gave way to European-style drugs. However, in certain regions such as Appalachia, Alaska,

Hawaii, and remote tribal lands in the western United States and Canada, herbal medicine continues to be widely relied upon.

South America

Medicinal plants were widely utilized by the indigenous populations of Central and South America. Shamanic traditions are still practiced today, utilizing the same plant medicines that have been highly regarded for centuries. This continent is abundant in plants that have numerous medicinal properties. Traditional healers, known as yerbaristes, can be found selling their remedies at market stalls. Forest workers often spend extended periods in the jungle, depending on plants for sustenance, healing remedies, and materials for constructing shelters.

The vast herbal knowledge that still exists in remote jungle locations is truly remarkable. Ancient Mayan and Aztec healers were well-versed in the use of various treatments derived from healing plants. In addition, they operated hospitals where individuals in need of medical care were provided with dedicated attention and isolated from the general population.

Today, South American land is now occupied by cities, plantations, and ranches, leaving behind the once vibrant native flora. However, South America is home to a vast array of medicinal plants within its dense jungles. Exciting new species are constantly being discovered, underscoring the importance of conservation efforts and offering hope for breakthrough treatments in areas such as malaria and cancer.

Note

This book empowers you to take control of your health, while acknowledging the importance of modern medical care. Use these treatments with caution and discretion. If you have a persistent medical condition, it is advisable to consult a doctor.

Chapter 2

The Scientific Basis behind the Remedies

We've discovered that numerous herbs and botanicals serve as the foundation for several widely-used medications. As we delve into the remedies, we'll discuss this in more depth, but here's a fundamental explanation of how herbal remedies function.

Gastrointestinal Health and Good Liver Function

Herbal remedies can be effective in addressing minor digestive complaints like indigestion and nausea. A cup of peppermint or chamomile tea can be quite soothing and help you feel more at ease.

Even livers that are overwhelmed can benefit from the use of certain herbs, which offer protection and aid in restoring normal function after injury or illness.

Milk thistle is a widely recognized herb that promotes liver health.

Immune Function, Infection, and Inflammation

Several botanical medicines have the potential to enhance your immune system and aid in preventing infections and reducing inflammation. Echinacea is a fantastic immune-stimulant herb that aids in infection prevention, while ginseng is a botanical that can enhance the immune system and support overall well-being. St. John's wort, ginger, and ginkgo biloba are excellent botanicals known for their anti-inflammatory properties.

Musculoskeletal Discomfort

Internal and external herbal medicines can effectively address minor sprains, sore muscles, and painful joints. Botanicals that are rich in antioxidants work wonders for maintaining the health of connective tissues. On the outside, the soothing properties of herbs such as calendula, witch hazel, and capsicum provide a comforting experience.

Psychological, Neurological, and Behavioral Health

When you watch an advertisement for prescription drugs that aim to improve mental health, it becomes apparent that most of them include warnings about potential side effects. Herbal remedies such as ginkgo biloba and valerian have the potential to restore balance without any negative side effects.

Reproductive Health

Knowing which herbs to use can make managing premenstrual syndrome (PMS), menopause symptoms, and pregnancy side effects easier. Ginger is effective in managing morning sickness, while black cohosh is known to alleviate symptoms of both PMS and menopause. Herbs like ginseng, ginkgo biloba, and saw palmetto can be beneficial for supporting the male reproductive system.

Respiratory Health

Common ailments like sore throats, coughs, and colds can be alleviated with the help of readily available medications, although they may sometimes come with unpleasant side effects. Nevertheless, these annoyances can be effectively addressed with herbal remedies, just like congested sinuses and mild respiratory infections. Echinacea is commonly used in cold and flu treatments, while thyme and hyssop are known for their ability to relieve bronchial spasms and promote rest.

Chapter 3

Remedies and Recipes

Everyday ailments can be easily treated with basic recipes, simple kitchen tools, and a well-stocked pharmacy of herbs. Whether you have experienced the discomfort of a bee sting while tending to your tomatoes or the unfortunate incident of being hit by a flying baseball at your child's Little League game, you will discover a comprehensive list of helpful remedies here.

Abscess

An abscess can be quite uncomfortable and may feel warm when touched. It occurs when an area becomes inflamed or infected and fills with pus. The pain of an abscess intensifies as it grows larger. If herbal remedies are not effective, it is important to seek medical attention as the infection within a large abscess can potentially spread to the surrounding tissue and even enter the bloodstream.

Fresh Yarrow Poultice

Makes I poultice

Yarrow possesses compounds with anti-inflammatory and antibacterial properties. It effectively eliminates bacteria, reduces inflammation, and accelerates the healing process.

Ingredients

I tablespoon of finely chopped fresh yarrow leaves.

Steps

Use the chopped leaves to treat the abscess, and make sure to cover it with a soft cloth. Keep the poultice in place for 10 to 15 minutes.

Continue this routine two or three times per day until the abscess has fully healed.

Precautions Do not use during pregnancy. Yarrow can cause skin reactions in people who are allergic to plants in the Asteraceae family.

Echinacea and Goldenseal Tincture

Makes about 2 cups

Echinacea and goldenseal provide powerful antibacterial benefits and enhance your body's natural immune response. Prepare this tincture in advance to ensure it's readily available when required. When stored in an optimal environment, it can maintain its quality for a duration of 7 years. Feel free to utilize it whenever you encounter an infection.

Ingredients

5 ounces dried echinacea root, finely chopped

3 ounces dried goldenseal root, finely chopped

2 cups unflavored 80-proof vodkatttt

Steps

Combine the echinacea and goldenseal in a sterilized pint jar. Ensure that the vodka is added generously, filling the jar to its maximum capacity and ensuring that the herbs are fully submerged.

Make sure to secure the jar firmly and give it a good shake. Keep it in a cool, dark cabinet and give it a gentle shake every few days for 6 to 8 weeks. If any of the alcohol evaporates, make sure to replenish it with more vodka until the jar is once again filled to the brim.

Moisten a piece of cheesecloth and carefully place it over the opening of a funnel. Transfer the tincture through the funnel into a clean pint jar. Extract the liquid from the roots by firmly squeezing the cheesecloth until all the liquid has been released. Dispose of the roots and pour the completed tincture into glass bottles of a dark color.

For the treatment of an abscess, it is recommended to take 10 drops orally two or three times a day for a duration of 7 to 10 days.

Precautions Do not use during pregnancy. Use caution if you have diabetes, as goldenseal can sometimes lower blood sugar.

Acne

Painful pimples are caused by sebaceous glands that are red, inflamed, and infected. Although this condition typically impacts teenagers, adults are also susceptible to it. Whether acne is limited to your face or has extended to your chest, back, or other areas of your body, herbal remedies can assist in improving your appearance and overall well-being.

Calendula Toner

Makes about ½ cup

This simple toner contains soothing calendula to address inflammation and witch hazel to target bacteria while softening your skin. When stored in an optimal environment, this toner maintains its freshness for a minimum of one year.

Ingredients

2 tablespoons calendula oil

⅓ cup witch hazel

Steps

Mix the ingredients together in a glass bottle and give it a gentle shake.
Using a cotton cosmetic pad, gently apply 5 or 6 drops to your clean face or any areas that require attention. Adjust the amount as necessary.
Continue using twice daily until acne clears. If you desire a refreshing experience, consider storing the bottle in the refrigerator.

Agrimony-Chamomile Gel

Makes about ⅔ cup

Combining agrimony and chamomile with aloe vera gel can provide relief from redness and inflammation. It is recommended to store the gel in the refrigerator. When stored in a sealed container, it will stay fresh for up to 2 weeks.

Ingredients

2 teaspoons dried agrimony

2 teaspoons dried chamomile

½ cup water

¼ cup aloe vera gel

Steps

Combine the agrimony and chamomile with the water in a saucepan. Bring the mixture to a boil over high heat, then lower the heat to a gentle simmer. Let the mixture simmer until it is reduced by half, then take it off the heat and let it cool completely.

Moisten a piece of cheesecloth and place it over the opening of a funnel. Transfer the mixture through the funnel into a glass bowl. Extract the liquid from the herbs, firmly squeezing the cheesecloth until no more liquid is left.

Mix the aloe vera gel with the liquid using a whisk until well blended. Transfer the finished gel to a clean glass jar. Make sure to seal the jar securely and place it in the refrigerator.

Using a cotton cosmetic pad, gently apply a thin layer to the affected areas twice a day.

Precautions Omit the chamomile if you take prescription blood thinners or are allergic to plants in the ragweed family

Allergies

Allergies manifest as atypical immune reactions to everyday substances like cat dander, pollen, or dust. Allergens can be found in various sources such as food, drinks, and the environment, making it challenging to completely avoid them. While traditional treatments may suppress the immune response to allergens, herbal remedies offer a more gentle approach.

Feverfew-Peppermint Tincture

Makes about 2 cups

Feverfew and peppermint can help to open up the airways when experiencing an allergy attack. If you prefer to avoid feverfew, you can create a tincture using only peppermint. The tincture can be stored for a maximum of 7 years in a cool, dark location.

Ingredients

2 ounces dried feverfew

6 ounces dried peppermint

2 cups unflavored 80-proof vodka

Steps

Combine the feverfew and peppermint in a sterilized pint jar. Please add the vodka, ensuring that the jar is filled to its maximum capacity.

Make sure to securely seal the jar and give it a good shake. Keep it in a cool, dark cabinet and give it a gentle shake a few times each week for 6 to 8 weeks.

Moisten a piece of cheesecloth and place it gently over the opening of a funnel. Transfer the tincture through the funnel into a clean pint jar. Squeeze out the liquid from the herbs. Dispose of the used herbs and pour the completed tincture into glass bottles of a dark color.

Administer 5 drops orally as needed when allergy symptoms arise. If the flavor is too intense for your liking, you have the option to dilute it by mixing it with a glass of water or juice before consumption.

Precautions Do not use feverfew if you are allergic to ragweed. Do not use feverfew during pregnancy.

Garlic-Ginkgo Syrup

Makes about 2 cups

Ginkgo biloba is a natural antihistamine that has numerous anti-inflammatory properties, while garlic can strengthen your immune system. If available, opt for locally sourced honey, as it can enhance your resistance to allergens in your vicinity. This syrup can remain fresh for up to 6 months when stored in the refrigerator.

Ingredients

2 ounces fresh or freeze-dried garlic, chopped

2 ounces ginkgo biloba, crushed or chopped

2 cups water

1 cup local honey

Steps

In a saucepan, combine the garlic and ginkgo biloba with the water. Heat the liquid gently until it simmers, then partially cover with a lid and let it reduce by half.

Pour the contents of the saucepan into a glass measuring cup. Then, strain the mixture back into the saucepan using a dampened piece of cheesecloth. Squeeze the cheesecloth until no more liquid is released.

Include the honey and gently heat the mixture on low, stirring continuously and ceasing when the temperature reaches 105°F to 110°F.

Transfer the syrup to a sterilized jar or bottle and keep it in the refrigerator.

Take 1 tablespoon by mouth three times daily until your allergy symptoms improve.

Safety Measures Caution: Avoid use if you are currently taking a monoamine oxidase inhibitor (MAOI) for depression. It is important to consult with your doctor before using Ginkgo biloba, as it can potentially enhance the effects of blood thinners. For optimal results, it is recommended that children under the age of 12 take 1 teaspoon three times per day.

Asthma

This condition is characterized by irritated airways throughout the lungs, as well as narrowed bronchial tubes. Experiencing difficulty in breathing can be quite terrifying for individuals, leading to potential panic attacks.

Ginkgo-Thyme Tea

Makes I cup

Ginkgo biloba and thyme can assist in opening your airways and promoting relaxation in the chest muscles, resulting in improved breathing. If the taste of this tea is not to your liking, consider enhancing it with a teaspoon of honey or dried peppermint to enhance its flavor.

Ingredients

I cup boiling water

I teaspoon dried ginkgo biloba

I teaspoon dried thyme

Steps

Fill a big mug with boiling water. Put in the dried herbs, cover the mug, and let the tea steep for 10 minutes. Take it easy and savor the tea while breathing in the steam. You can do this up to four times a day.

Peppermint-Rosemary Vapor Treatment

Makes I treatment

Peppermint can assist in opening up your airways and promoting easier breathing, while rosemary leaves contain a beneficial oil that can block histamine. If fresh herbs are not available for this treatment, they can be substituted with 2 drops of peppermint essential oil and 4 drops of rosemary essential oil.

Ingredients

4 cups steaming-hot water (not boiling)

½ cup crushed fresh peppermint leaves

½ cup finely chopped fresh rosemary leaves

Steps

Combine all the ingredients in a large, shallow bowl. Position the bowl on a table and settle yourself comfortably in front of it.

Place a generous-sized towel over your head and the bowl. Experience the intoxicating aroma of the herbal vapors. Take breaks as necessary to get some fresh air, and if the fumes become overwhelming, simply close your eyes. Keep up with the treatment until the water has cooled down.

Use as necessary whenever asthma symptoms occur. This treatment is gentle enough to use as frequently as you prefer.

Athlete's Foot

This uncomfortable infection is caused by a fungus that prefers moist, warm, dark environments. Make sure to address the issue before it spreads to your toenails, as it can lead to unsightly discoloration and disfigurement that can be challenging to eliminate.

Fresh Garlic Poultice

Makes I treatment

Garlic is an incredibly potent antifungal agent that effectively eliminates athlete's foot. Using raw honey can help bind the garlic to your feet and enhance its antifungal properties. If you want to speed up the healing process, it's recommended to make a fresh batch of this remedy for each treatment. While it's possible to make a larger quantity and use it over a few days, using a fresh batch each time may yield faster results.

Ingredients

I garlic clove, pressed

I teaspoon raw honey

Steps

Combine the garlic and honey in a small bowl. Using a cotton cosmetic pad, gently apply the blend to the affected area. Slip into a fresh pair of socks and take a moment to unwind, allowing the poultice to work its magic for 15 minutes to an hour. Make sure to wash and dry your feet thoroughly afterwards. Continue the treatment once or twice per day, and then apply Goldenseal Ointment as directed. Continue for three days after symptoms have resolved.

Precautions Garlic may cause a skin rash in sensitive individuals.

Goldenseal Ointment

Makes about I cup

Goldenseal is a powerful antimicrobial agent that effectively combats athlete's foot. You have the option to use this ointment alone or enhance its healing properties by combining it with a Fresh Garlic Poultice. When stored in a cool, dark place, it will remain fresh for up to a year.

Ingredients

I cup light olive oil

2 ounces dried goldenseal root, chopped

I ounce beeswax

Steps

Combine the olive oil and goldenseal in a slow cooker. Choose the lowest heat setting, cover the slow cooker, and let the roots steep in the oil for 3 to 5 hours. Disable the heat and let the infused oil cool down.

Bring a small amount of water to a gentle simmer in the base of a double boiler.

Lower the heat to a lower setting.

Place a piece of cheesecloth over the top half of the double boiler. Add the infused oil and squeeze the cheesecloth tightly to extract all the oil. Dispose of the cheesecloth and used herbs.

Combine the beeswax with the infused oil and carefully position the double boiler on the base.

Warm the mixture gently over low heat. Once the beeswax has completely melted, carefully take the pan off the heat. Efficiently transfer the mixture into clean, dry jars or tins and ensure it cools completely before sealing.

Using a cotton cosmetic pad, gently apply a small amount to the areas that need attention. Adjust the amount as necessary and apply up to three times daily, with the last application before bedtime. It is recommended to wear a pair of clean socks over the ointment to prevent any potential slipping.

Precautions Do not use if you are pregnant or breastfeeding. Do not use if you have high blood pressure.

Backache

Although back pain is often a result of overwork or injury, it can also be caused by inactivity, muscle spasms, or inflammation. Take the time to rest as much as possible in order to promote healing. If you experience intense pain or notice any symptoms such as numbness, tingling, or incontinence, it is important to consult with your doctor.

Passionflower–Blue Vervain Tea

Makes I cup

Passionflower and blue vervain have calming effects on the nervous system and can provide relief for tense muscles. This blend is incredibly soothing, so make sure to enjoy it when you have a moment to unwind.

Ingredients

I cup boiling water

I teaspoon dried passionflower

I teaspoon dried blue vervain

Steps

Transfer the hot water into a spacious mug. Include the dried herbs, place a lid on the mug, and let the tea steep for 10 minutes. Take your time and savor the tea. Can be repeated up to two times daily

Precautions Do not use passionflower or blue vervain during pregnancy. Avoid passionflower if you have prostate problems or baldness.

Ginger-Peppermint Salve

Makes about I cup

Ginger and peppermint have powerful properties that can deeply penetrate the skin, resulting in a soothing and comforting feeling that helps to relax the muscles. This salve will stay fresh for up to a year if stored in a cool, dark place.

Ingredients

I cup light olive oil

I ounce dried gingerroot, chopped

I ounce dried peppermint, crushed

I ounce beeswax

Steps

Combine the olive oil, ginger, and peppermint in a slow cooker. Choose the lowest heat setting, cover the slow cooker, and let the herbs steep in the oil for 3 to 5 hours. Switch off the heat and let the infused oil cool down.

Bring a small amount of water to a gentle simmer in the base of a double boiler.

Lower the heat to a gentle simmer.

Place a piece of cheesecloth over the top portion of the double boiler. Add the infused oil and squeeze the cheesecloth tightly until all the oil has been extracted. Dispose of the cheesecloth and used herbs.

Combine the beeswax with the infused oil and carefully position the double boiler on the base.

Warm slowly over low heat. Once the beeswax has melted completely, carefully take the pan off the heat. Efficiently transfer the mixture into pristine, moisture-free jars or tins and let it cool entirely before sealing.

Apply I teaspoon of the product to the affected area and massage it in using your fingers or a cotton cosmetic pad. Adjust the amount as necessary. Continue the treatment up to four times per day.

Bee Sting

It is common to experience pain, redness, and swelling after being stung by a bee, and these symptoms can persist for a while. Herbs can provide relief from discomfort. However, it's important to note that while herbal treatments can be beneficial, they should not be relied upon as a substitute for emergency EpiPens, especially if you have an allergy to bee venom.

Fresh Plantain Poultice

Makes I treatment

The plantain plant, distinct from the banana, is a green weed that contains aucubin, a powerful antitoxin.

Other components provide antiseptic and anti-inflammatory advantages, enhancing the effectiveness of this straightforward treatment. If fresh plantain leaves are not available, you can rehydrate a teaspoon of dried, crushed plantain in a tablespoon of water to use as a poultice.

Ingredients

I tablespoon finely chopped fresh plantain leaves

Steps

Place the chopped leaves on the affected area and gently cover it with a soft cloth. Keep the poultice on for 10 to 15 minutes. Repeat as often as necessary until the pain subsides permanently.

Comfrey-Aloe Gel

Makes about ¼ cup

Comfrey has remarkable anti-inflammatory and analgesic properties that can provide relief from the pain and swelling caused by bee stings. Aloe offers a soothing sensation and accelerates the healing process. If you enjoy this balm, you'll discover its usefulness for a range of minor cuts and scrapes. When stored in the refrigerator, it remains fresh for approximately 2 weeks.

Ingredients

2 teaspoons dried comfrey

¼ cup water

2 tablespoons aloe vera gel

Steps

Combine the comfrey and water in a saucepan. Bring the mixture to a boil over high heat, then lower the heat to a gentle simmer. Cook the mixture until it reduces by half, then take it off the heat and let it cool completely.

Moisten a piece of cheesecloth and carefully place it over the opening of a funnel. Transfer the mixture through the funnel into a glass bowl. Extract the liquid from the comfrey by firmly squeezing the cheesecloth until all the liquid has been released.

Combine the aloe vera gel with the liquid and mix thoroughly using a whisk. Place the completed gel into a sterilized glass jar. Make sure to seal the jar securely and place it in the refrigerator.

Using a cotton cosmetic pad, gently apply a thin layer to the affected area whenever necessary until the pain and swelling decrease.

Bloating

Indulging in excessive food, experiencing abdominal gas, and the arrival of women's premenstrual cycles are some factors that can trigger an unpleasant episode of bloating. Herbs assist in restoring your body's equilibrium by aiding in the removal of toxins, excessive gas, and accumulated fluid.

Peppermint-Fennel Tea

Makes I cup

If you think that your bloating may be due to buildup in your digestive tract, peppermint and fennel can offer you comfort and fast relief. These plants have a delightful taste and contain powerful antispasmodic agents that help to relax the smooth muscle tissue in the digestive tract. If the flavor of this tea is too strong for you, consider adding a teaspoon of honey.

Ingredients

I cup boiling water

I teaspoon dried peppermint

¼ teaspoon fennel seeds, crushed

Steps

Transfer the hot water into a spacious mug. Include the peppermint and fennel, place a lid on the mug, and let the tea steep for 10 minutes.

Take a moment to unwind and savor your cup of tea. This remedy is gentle and can be used as frequently as necessary.

Dandelion Root Tincture

Makes about 2 cups

Dandelion root has a bitter taste, but it provides potent diuretic benefits that can aid in the elimination of toxins and promote a greater sense of comfort. This tincture can maintain its freshness for a remarkable 7 years when stored in a cool, dark place.

Ingredients

8 ounces dandelion root, finely chopped

2 cups unflavored 80-proof vodka

Steps

Place the dandelion root into a sterilized pint jar. Ensure that the vodka is added generously, filling the jar to its utmost capacity and ensuring that the roots are fully submerged.

Make sure to seal the jar securely and give it a good shake. Keep it in a cool, dark cabinet and give it a good shake a few times each week for 6 to 8 weeks. If any of the alcohol evaporates, simply add more vodka to fill the jar to the brim once again.

Moisten a piece of cheesecloth and carefully place it over the opening of a funnel. Transfer the tincture through the funnel into a clean pint jar. Extract the liquid from the roots by firmly squeezing the cheesecloth until all the liquid has been released. Dispose of the roots and transfer the completed tincture into glass bottles of a dark color.

Take I teaspoon orally once or twice per day whenever bloating is a concern. If the flavor is too intense for your liking, you have the option to dilute it by mixing it with a glass of water or juice before consumption.

Bronchitis

Bronchitis is commonly caused by irritation, infection, or allergies, leading to inflammation of the bronchial linings. The condition is typically accompanied by a deep, rasping cough. Herbal treatments, along with a focus on staying hydrated and getting ample rest, have been found to be effective in alleviating and getting rid of the symptoms of bronchitis.

Rosemary–Licorice Root Vapor Treatment

Makes 1 treatment

Rosemary and licorice root can assist in opening the airways, promoting circulation, and providing relief from the discomfort and inflammation commonly associated with bronchitis.

Ingredients

5 cups water

¼ cup chopped dried licorice root

½ cup finely chopped fresh rosemary leaves

Steps

Combine the water and dried licorice root in a saucepan. Heat the mixture until it boils, then lower the heat. Cook gently for 10 minutes.

Combine the water and licorice root in a shallow bowl, then incorporate the rosemary leaves.

Place a generously-sized towel over your head and the bowl. Inhale the fragrant vapors that gently waft from the herbs. Take breaks as necessary to get some fresh air, and if the fumes become overwhelming, simply close your eyes. Keep the treatment going until the water has cooled down.

Repeat as necessary. This treatment can be used as frequently as desired without causing any harm.

Precautions Do not use this treatment if you have epilepsy, high blood pressure, diabetes, kidney problems, or heart disease.

Goldenseal-Hyssop Syrup

Makes about 2 cups

Goldenseal is known for its powerful antiviral and antibacterial properties, thanks to the presence of hydrastine and berberine. Hyssop is known for its ability to alleviate bronchial spasms and promote the clearance of lung congestion. Additionally, it has a soothing and calming effect that can assist in relaxation. This syrup is also effective in treating the common cold. It can be stored in the refrigerator for up to 6 months.

Ingredients

½ ounce dried goldenseal root, chopped

I ounce dried hyssop

2 cups water

I cup honey

Steps

Combine the goldenseal and hyssop with the water in a saucepan. Heat the liquid gently until it simmers, then partially cover with a lid and let it reduce by half.

Pour the contents of the saucepan into a glass measuring cup, and then strain the mixture through a dampened piece of cheesecloth back into the saucepan. Squeeze the cheesecloth until all the liquid has been extracted.

Incorporate the honey and gently heat the mixture on a low flame, ensuring to stir consistently until the temperature reaches 105°F to 110°F.

Transfer the syrup into a sterilized jar or bottle and keep it in the refrigerator.

Take 1 tablespoon orally three to five times per day until your symptoms improve.

Precautions: Avoid usage during pregnancy or while breastfeeding. Caution: Not recommended for individuals with epilepsy or high blood pressure. Goldenseal may worsen symptoms of diarrhea and heartburn. For children under age 12, it is recommended to take 1 teaspoon two to three times per day.

Bruise

Deep, painful bruises may suggest the presence of other injuries or health complications. Minor bruises can result from accidental contact with objects. If you notice an increase in the frequency of bruising, it is advisable to consult with your doctor, as this could potentially indicate an underlying health concern.

Fresh Hyssop Poultice

Makes 1 treatment

Hyssop provides pain relief and promotes circulation, which can accelerate the healing process of your bruise. If you haven't already incorporated hyssop into your garden, you can utilize a small amount of hyssop essential oil to address a bruise. Another option is to rehydrate a teaspoon of dried hyssop with a tablespoon of warm water and use it to make a poultice.

Ingredients

1 tablespoon finely chopped fresh hyssop leaves

Steps

Place the chopped leaves on the affected area and gently cover it with a soft cloth. Keep the poultice in place for 10 to 15 minutes. Continue this routine two or three times daily until the bruise gradually disappears.

Precautions Hyssop can produce sudden and involuntary muscle contractions, so it should not be used if you have epilepsy or are pregnant.

Arnica Salve

Makes about 1 cup

Arnica is a powerful anti-inflammatory agent, and its pain-relieving properties make this simple salve a great option for bumps and bruises.

Ingredients

I cup light olive oil

2 ounces dried arnica flowers

I ounce beeswax

Steps

Combine the olive oil and arnica in a slow cooker. Choose the lowest heat setting, cover the slow cooker, and let the herbs steep in the oil for 3 to 5 hours. Disable the heat and let the infused oil cool down.

Heat a small amount of water in the base of a double boiler until it simmers.

Lower the heat to a lower setting.

Place a piece of cheesecloth gently over the upper half of the double boiler. Add the infused oil and squeeze the cheesecloth tightly to extract all the oil. Dispose of the cheesecloth and used herbs.

Combine the beeswax with the infused oil and carefully position the double boiler on the base.

Warm slowly over low heat. Once the beeswax has melted completely, carefully take the pan off the heat. Pour the mixture into clean, dry jars or tins and let it cool completely before sealing.

Using your fingers or a cotton cosmetic pad, gently apply a small amount to the affected area. Adjust the amount as necessary and apply twice daily until the bruise diminishes.

Precautions: Do not use on broken skin. Irritation can occur with long-term use; discontinue if signs of skin irritation appear.

Burn

Herbal remedies are effective for minor burns, like those that can happen while cooking. It is crucial to promptly seek medical attention for burns that appear to be severe, with charred skin or extensive coverage on the body.

Chickweed-Mullein Compress

Makes I treatment

Mullein has properties that can help prevent burns from getting infected and provide relief from pain.

Chickweed offers an extra level of cooling and aids in expediting the healing process.

Ingredients

2 teaspoons finely chopped chickweed

I teaspoon finely chopped fresh mullein leaf

Steps

Apply the freshly cut plant material to the burn and the area around it, then cover it with a gentle cloth. Keep the poultice on for 10 to 15 minutes. Continue the repetition every 2 to 3 hours or more frequently, until the pain diminishes.

Fresh Aloe Vera Gel

Makes I treatment

Aloe vera gel has powerful antibacterial properties that effectively protect burns from infection. Additionally, it provides soothing anti-inflammatory benefits. Aloe has the ability to stimulate collagen synthesis, which can help accelerate the regeneration process of the skin following a minor burn. Although it is most effective when used immediately after being extracted from the plant, bottled aloe gel can be a suitable alternative.

Ingredients

Aloe vera plant

Steps

Take a 1-inch section from the tip of an aloe vera leaf. Keep the remaining leaf on the plant to support its ongoing growth.

Using a precise knife, carefully cut the leaf open. Apply the gel from the center of the leaf to the burn and the surrounding area using your fingers or a cotton cosmetic pad. Make sure to repeat this process once or twice a day while your burn is healing.

Canker Sore

An occasional canker sore, a painful red blister that mysteriously appears inside the mouth, can be quite irritating but is generally not a cause for concern. It is advisable to consult with a healthcare professional if canker sores occur frequently, as they may be a sign of an underlying metabolic disorder.

Calendula-Comfrey Poultice

Makes I treatment

Calendula is known for its soothing properties and ability to promote faster healing of minor wounds. It also has antifungal, anti-inflammatory, and antibacterial benefits. Comfrey is known for its healing properties and can provide some relief from the pain and itching associated with canker sores. If you enjoy this treatment, you can optimize your time by creating multiple dry poultices simultaneously.

Ingredients

⅛ teaspoon dried calendula

⅛ teaspoon dried comfrey

2 tablespoons hot water

Steps

Utilize a mortar and pestle or grinder to finely grind the herbs, then carefully transfer the resulting powder onto a small piece of muslin fabric.

Carefully fold the muslin into a compact packet, making sure to enclose the fragrant herbs. Immerse it in hot water for 2 minutes.

Insert the completed poultice into your mouth, ensuring that the fabric layer is thin and in contact with the canker sore. Keep it in place for 10 to 15 minutes. Repeat the process two or three times per day until the canker sore is gone.

Goldenseal Tincture

Makes about ⅔ cup

Goldenseal root contains berberine and hydrastine, making it a valuable herb with broad-spectrum antiviral and antibacterial properties. In addition to using this goldenseal tincture for canker sores, it can also be used to treat minor cuts, scrapes, and burns. You can also consume it internally when you sense the onset of a cold or the flu.

Ingredients

4 ounces dried goldenseal root, finely chopped

1 cup unflavored 80-proof vodka

Steps

Place the goldenseal in a sanitized half-pint jar. Fill the jar to the brim with vodka, ensuring that the roots are completely covered.

Make sure to seal the jar securely and give it a good shake. Keep it in a cool, dark cabinet and give it a good shake a few times each week for 6 to 8 weeks. If any of the alcohol evaporates, make sure to replenish it with more vodka until the jar is filled to the brim once again.

Moisten a piece of cheesecloth and carefully place it over the opening of a funnel. Transfer the tincture through the funnel into a clean, sterilized half-pint jar. Extract the liquid from the roots by firmly squeezing the cheesecloth until all the liquid has been wrung out. Remove the roots and carefully transfer the completed tincture into glass bottles that are dark in color.

Apply 2 or 3 drops on the canker sore using a cotton swab. Inhale through your mouth to prevent excessive saliva while the tincture dries. Continue using this method two or three times per day until the canker sore goes away.

Precautions: Not recommended for use during pregnancy or while breastfeeding. Do not use if you have high blood pressure.

Chapped Lips

At times, lips can become painfully cracked or rough and peeling, which is more than just a cosmetic issue. Dryness of the lips can often occur when they are unable to naturally produce moisture. Exposure to sun, wind, heating, and air-conditioning can exacerbate the situation, as can licking your lips in an attempt to moisturize them and alleviate any discomfort you may be experiencing.

Aloe-Calendula Balm

Makes 2 tablespoons

Aloe vera and calendula are beneficial for healing compromised skin, while aloe provides much-needed moisture to dry lips. This recipe utilizes a ready-made calendula oil, but feel free to substitute it with your own homemade infused calendula oil. When properly stored, this balm will remain fresh for up to a year.

Ingredients

I ½ tablespoons aloe vera gel

I ½ teaspoons calendula oil

Steps

Combine the aloe vera gel and calendula oil in a small bowl. Make sure to blend them thoroughly with a whisk.

Move the balm to a container that has a secure lid. If you want to ensure the freshness of your main supply, it's recommended to keep it refrigerated. However, you may also consider carrying a small squeeze bottle with a teaspoon of it to conveniently apply throughout the day.

Using either your fingertip or a cotton swab, gently apply a thin layer to your lips. Only a small amount is necessary, apply as necessary during the day and before going to sleep.

Comfrey-Hyssop Lip Balm

Makes about ⅔ cup (enough to fill 10 lip balm tubes)

Both comfrey and hyssop have properties that can reduce inflammation and pain, which can help speed up the healing process of damaged skin and provide some relief from the discomfort of chapped lips. This recipe can be easily adjusted to make more or less servings. The final product will remain fresh for approximately one year if stored in a cool, dark location.

Ingredients

2 tablespoons jojoba oil

1 tablespoon cocoa butter

1 tablespoon light olive oil

1 teaspoon dried comfrey

1 teaspoon dried hyssop

4 teaspoons grated beeswax or beeswax pastilles

3 drops vitamin E oil (optional)

Steps

Bring a small amount of water to a gentle simmer in the base of a double boiler.

Lower the heat to a low setting.

Combine the jojoba oil, cocoa butter, olive oil, and herbs in a glass measuring cup. Position the measuring cup in the top section of the double boiler and let it warm slowly over low heat for a duration of 2 to 3 hours. Remember to regularly monitor the water level in the base of the double boiler to prevent any potential evaporation.

Place a small bowl and cover it with a layer of cheesecloth. Carefully strain the infused oil into the bowl. Squeeze and wring the cheesecloth until all the oil has been extracted.

Dispose of the cheesecloth and used herbs.

Place the infused oil back into the measuring cup and incorporate the beeswax. Place the measuring cup back on the top of the double boiler and warm it over low heat until the beeswax has melted, being careful not to apply too much heat.

Take out the measuring cup from the double boiler and include the vitamin E oil (if desired). Pour the mixture into clean, dry lip balm tubes or tins and let it cool completely before capping.

Remember to regularly apply a thin layer of balm to your lips during the day and before bedtime for optimal results.

Precautions: Omit the hyssop and double the comfrey if you are pregnant or have epilepsy.

Chest Congestion

If you're experiencing difficulty breathing, herbs can provide relief for your lungs and enhance your comfort as you work towards resolving the underlying cause of your congestion.

Hyssop-Sage Infusion

Makes 1 quart

Hyssop has powerful antiviral properties and is known for its effectiveness as an expectorant. Sage has beneficial antiseptic properties that can aid in faster healing. This blend offers a robust herbal flavor that appeals to certain individuals, while others may prefer to enhance its palatability by adding a touch of honey.

Ingredients

4 cups boiling water

4 teaspoons dried hyssop

4 teaspoons dried sage

Steps

Combine the boiling water and dried herbs in a teapot. Cover the pot and let the infusion steep for 10 minutes.

Take a moment to unwind and savor the soothing aroma as you leisurely sip on your infusion. You have the option to reheat or refrigerate the remaining portion and enjoy it throughout the day.

Angelica-Goldenseal Syrup

Makes about 2 cups

Angelica helps to relieve congestion by gently stimulating and warming the lungs, providing relief from associated discomfort. Goldenseal has powerful antiseptic and antiviral properties, which can assist in speeding up your recovery from illness. Honey masks the strong flavors while soothing your throat, which may feel a bit irritated from any coughing. This syrup will remain fresh for up to 6 months when stored in the refrigerator.

Ingredients

1 ounce angelica, finely chopped

1 ounce dried goldenseal root, finely chopped

2 cups water

1 cup honey

Steps

Combine the herbs and water in a saucepan. Simmer the liquid over low heat, partially covering it with a lid, until it is reduced by half.

Transfer the contents of the saucepan to a glass measuring cup, then pour the mixture through a dampened piece of cheesecloth back into the saucepan, squeezing the cheesecloth until no more liquid is extracted.

Include the honey and gently heat the mixture on a low flame, stirring continuously until the temperature reaches 105°F to 110°F.

Transfer the syrup to a sterilized jar or bottle and keep it in the refrigerator.

Take 1 tablespoon orally three or four times per day until your symptoms improve. For children under age 12, it is recommended to take 1 teaspoon two or three times per day.

Chicken Pox

An extremely contagious infection, chicken pox causes a rash that is itchy and filled with blisters. While there is no cure for chicken pox, utilizing herbal remedies can provide some relief from the discomfort.

Comfrey-Licorice Bath

Makes I quart

Comfrey and licorice root provide relief for the itching caused by chicken pox and also have antiviral properties. The apple cider vinegar has a strong aroma, but it enhances the soothing effect. This simple recipe utilizes pre-made comfrey and licorice root tinctures, although you have the option to substitute them with your own homemade versions.

Ingredients

4 cups organic unfiltered apple cider vinegar

½ teaspoon comfrey tincture

½ teaspoon licorice root tincture

Steps

Combine the vinegar and tinctures in a clean, dry jar. Seal tightly and keep in a cool, dark place until you're ready to use it.

Prepare a warm bath and add I cup of the mixture to the water. Make sure to spend at least 20 minutes soaking. Make sure to repeat once or twice per day.

Precautions: Do not use licorice root if you have high blood pressure, diabetes, kidney problems, or heart disease.

Calendula-Goldenseal Gel

Makes about 2 cups

Aloe, calendula, and goldenseal work together to provide relief from itching and irritation, promoting the healing process of chicken pox blisters. This gel is excellent for treating various rashes and skin irritations, including minor cuts and scrapes. When refrigerated, it can stay fresh for up to 2 weeks.

Ingredients

I ounce dried calendula

I ounce dried goldenseal root, chopped

2 cups water

I ½ cups aloe vera gel

Steps

Combine the calendula and goldenseal with the water in a saucepan. Bring the mixture to a boil over high heat, then lower the heat to a gentle simmer.

Cook the mixture until only about ½ cup is left, then take it off the stove and let it cool completely.

Moisten a piece of cheesecloth and carefully place it over the opening of a funnel. Transfer the mixture through the funnel into a glass bowl. Extract the liquid from the herbs by firmly squeezing the cheesecloth until all the liquid has been released.

Combine the aloe vera gel with the liquid and mix using a whisk. Place the completed gel into a sterilized glass jar. Make sure to seal the jar securely and place it in the refrigerator.

Using a cotton cosmetic pad, gently apply a thin layer to the affected areas two or three times a day.

Cold

With symptoms that include coughing, sneezing, and a sore throat, the common cold can be a drag. Shorten your cold's duration by beginning treatment as soon as symptoms appear.

Thyme Tea

Makes 1 cup

Thyme has the ability to act as an antitussive, which means it can effectively suppress coughing and provide quick relief. It serves a dual purpose by helping to clear congestion from the lungs as an expectorant. Additionally, it provides relief for a sore throat and alleviates the body aches commonly experienced with a cold. If you prefer a sweeter flavor, you can add a teaspoon of honey to this tea.

Ingredients

1 cup boiling water

2 teaspoons dried thyme

Steps

Transfer the hot water into a spacious mug. Include the thyme, place a lid on the mug, and let the tea steep for 10 minutes.

Take your time and savor the tea as you enjoy the soothing aroma. Repeat up to six times per day.

Herbal Cold Syrup with Comfrey, Mullein, and Raspberry Leaf

Makes about 2 cups

Comfrey can be beneficial for coughs and sore throats, while mullein, thyme, and raspberry leaf have properties that can help with fever, body aches, and lung irritation. It's not a big deal if you're missing a couple of the herbs in this recipe. They all have beneficial properties that can help alleviate your cold symptoms. This syrup will remain fresh for up to 6 months when stored in the refrigerator.

Ingredients

½ ounce dried comfrey

½ ounce dried mullein

½ ounce dried raspberry leaf

½ ounce dried thyme

2 cups water

1 cup honey

Steps

Combine the herbs and water in a saucepan. Simmer the liquid gently over low heat, partially covering it with a lid, until it is reduced by half.

Pour the contents of the saucepan into a glass measuring cup. Then, strain the mixture back into the saucepan using a dampened piece of cheesecloth. Squeeze the cheesecloth until all the liquid has been extracted.

Include the honey and gently heat the mixture on low, stirring continuously until it reaches a temperature of 105°F to 110°F.

Transfer the syrup to a sterilized jar or bottle and keep it chilled in the refrigerator.

Take 1 tablespoon by mouth three or four times a day until your symptoms improve. For optimal results, it is recommended that children under the age of 12 take 1 teaspoon two or three times per day.

Precautions: Never use raspberry leaves that are not completely dried, as fresh ones can cause nausea

Cold Sore

Cold sores are a result of the herpes simplex virus and can be found in the mouth and on the lips. It is highly recommended to use herbal remedies as soon as you notice any tingling or itching, before the clusters of blisters appear.

If you happen to have an untreated cold sore, herbal remedies might not be potent enough to halt the virus's progression. However, they can offer comforting relief.

Garlic Poultice

Makes 1 treatment

Although raw garlic may have a strong smell, it possesses powerful antiviral properties that can potentially reduce the duration of a cold sore. If you prefer not to bother with holding the garlic in place, you might consider using a piece of first aid tape to secure it, allowing you to accomplish multiple tasks at once.

Ingredients

1 garlic clove, cut in half

Steps

Make sure to wash and dry the affected area thoroughly.

Place the cut side of the garlic on the cold sore and keep it there for 10 minutes. Continue this routine three or four times daily until the cold sore disappears.

Precautions: Garlic can cause a skin rash in sensitive individuals; discontinue treatment if this occurs.

Echinacea-Sage Toner

Makes about ½ cup

Echinacea and sage provide powerful antiviral and antibacterial properties, which can effectively prevent the sores from getting infected. The witch hazel and aloe are effective in providing relief from itching. This toner has a long shelf life of at least one year when stored in a refrigerator.

Ingredients

½ ounce dried echinacea root, chopped

½ ounce dried sage, crumbled

2 tablespoons jojoba or light olive oil

2 tablespoons aloe vera gel

¼ cup witch hazel

Steps

Combine the herbs and oil in a slow cooker. Choose the lowest heat setting, cover the slow cooker, and let the herbs steep in the oil for 3 to 5 hours.

Switch off the heat and let the infused oil cool down.

Place a piece of cheesecloth gently over a bowl. Strain the infused oil using the cheesecloth, making sure to squeeze out every last drop. Dispose of the cheesecloth and used herbs.

Place the infused oil into a glass bottle of a darker hue, and proceed to incorporate the aloe vera gel and witch hazel. Mix the ingredients by shaking gently.

Using a cotton swab, gently apply a small amount to the area that needs attention. Adjust the amount as necessary.

Continue using this method two or three times daily until the cold sore goes away. It is recommended to keep the bottle in the refrigerator.

Precautions: Omit the echinacea if you are allergic to ragweed or have an autoimmune disease.

Conjunctivitis

Symptoms of conjunctivitis include redness, itching, crusting or discharge, and tearing of the eyes. Also referred to as pinkeye, this common issue can result in dry eyes, swollen eyelids, and increased sensitivity to light.

Quick Chamomile Poultice

Makes I treatment

Chamomile is known for its soothing properties that can help alleviate the discomfort and irritation caused by conjunctivitis. It also has anti-inflammatory and antibacterial properties, making it a beneficial treatment option. Using plain chamomile tea bags, preferably organic, is a convenient and straightforward way to utilize this remedy when you're in a hurry.

Ingredients

¼ cup steaming-hot (not boiling) water

I organic chamomile tea bag

Steps

Place the water in a small cup or bowl and immerse the tea bag in it. Let it sit for 2 minutes.

Take out the tea bag from the water and let it cool down until it reaches a temperature that is warm and pleasant to touch. Take a moment to close your eye and find a state of relaxation. Gently press the tea bag against your eye and let it sit for 10 to 20 minutes. Replace two or three times per day while recovering from conjunctivitis.

Goldenseal Poultice

Makes 1 treatment

Goldenseal is highly effective in treating conjunctivitis due to its soothing properties that help reduce irritation, fight inflammation, and combat infection. If you enjoy this method, you can streamline the process by preparing multiple poultices ahead of time and simply activating them with hot water when you're ready to apply them.

Ingredients

½ cup steaming-hot water (not boiling)

1 tablespoon chopped dried goldenseal root

Steps

Transfer the hot water into a small bowl. Place the chopped goldenseal root in a reusable linen bag and submerge the bag in the hot water. Let the poultice soak in the water for 5 to 10 minutes, or until the roots become soft.

Take a moment to close your eyes and find a state of relaxation. Gently apply the poultice to your eye and let it sit for 10 to 20 minutes. Make sure to repeat two or three times per day while recovering from conjunctivitis.

Constipation

Abdominal discomfort and challenges with bowel movements are common signs of constipation. Herbs offer a gentle and effective way to find relief without the use of harsh chemical laxatives. Boost efficiency by increasing your fiber intake, staying hydrated, and being more physically active.

Aloe Vera Juice

Makes about 3 cups

Aloe vera juice enhances digestion and effectively cleanses the digestive tract. This makes it ideal for addressing long-term constipation issues. It is recommended to consume freshly made aloe juice within 3 days.

Ingredients

I fresh 3-to 4-inch aloe leaf from the inner portion of the plant

3 cups fresh juice, water, or coconut water

Steps

Flip the aloe leaf over the sink to let the resin drain away from the cut. Once the resin has stopped dripping, slice the leaf in half vertically and gently extract the gel from the interior. Transfer the gel to a blender and pour in the liquid. Blend thoroughly, refrigerate, and savor the refreshing result. Consume I cup daily and store any remaining mixture in a tightly sealed container in the refrigerator.

Dandelion-Chickweed Syrup

Makes about 2 cups

Both dandelion and chickweed are natural remedies that can help relieve constipation without the use of harsh chemicals. You might be able to find both of these herbs in your own backyard; just make sure that neither has been contaminated with herbicide or chemical fertilizer. This syrup will remain fresh for up to 6 months when stored in the refrigerator.

Ingredients

1 ounce dandelion root, chopped

1 ounce fresh or dried chickweed

2 cups water

1 cup honey

Steps

Combine the dandelion root, chickweed, and water in a saucepan. Bring the liquid to a gentle simmer over low heat, partially covering it with a lid, and allow the liquid to reduce by half.

Pour the contents of the saucepan into a glass measuring cup, and then strain the mixture back into the saucepan using a dampened piece of cheesecloth. Squeeze the cheesecloth until all the liquid has been extracted.

Incorporate the honey and gently heat the mixture on a low flame, ensuring to stir continuously until the temperature reaches 105°F to 110°F.

Transfer the syrup to a sterilized jar or bottle and keep it in the refrigerator.

Take I tablespoon orally three or four times per day until your symptoms improve. For children under age I2, it is recommended to take I teaspoon two or three times per day.

Cough

Coughing is a natural bodily response that helps to remove irritants and excess phlegm from the lungs and airways. Starting as a bothersome tickle in your throat, this can escalate into a more severe and persistent cough that is dry and unproductive. Herbal remedies can help in soothing sensitive throat tissues as you work on addressing the root cause.

Fennel-Hyssop Tea

Makes 1 cup

Fennel helps to loosen phlegm, which can make coughs more productive. If you're experiencing a dry, hacking cough and an irritated throat, you'll be pleased to know that this tea contains fennel and hyssop, which can provide fast relief from the discomfort.

Ingredients

1 cup boiling water

1 teaspoon fennel seeds

1 teaspoon dried hyssop

Steps

Transfer the hot water into a spacious mug. Add the herbs, cover the mug, and let the tea steep for 10 minutes.

Take your time and savor the tea as you enjoy the soothing steam. Can be repeated up to four times per day.

Licorice-Thyme Cough Syrup

Makes about 2 cups

Using licorice root can effectively reduce inflammation in the throat, providing fast relief for irritated tissue. Thyme, on the other hand, acts as an expectorant, helping to clear the lungs.

Thyme is also known for its antitussive properties, helping to soothe coughing spasms. This cough syrup has a shelf life of 6 months when stored in the refrigerator.

Ingredients

1 ounce licorice root, chopped

1 ounce thyme

2 cups water

1 cup honey

Steps

Combine the licorice root, thyme, and water in a saucepan. Heat the liquid gently until it simmers, then partially cover it with a lid and let it reduce by half.

Pour the contents of the saucepan into a glass measuring cup. Then, strain the mixture back into the saucepan using a dampened piece of cheesecloth, squeezing out all the liquid.

Incorporate the honey and gently heat the mixture on a low flame, ensuring to stir continuously until the temperature reaches 105°F to 110°F.

Transfer the syrup into a sterilized jar or bottle and keep it in the refrigerator.

Take 1 tablespoon orally three or four times per day until your symptoms improve. For optimal results, it is recommended that children under the age of 12 take 1 teaspoon two or three times per day.

Dandruff

Occasionally triggered by a fungal infection or scalp psoriasis, dandruff results in an uncomfortably itchy and flaky scalp. However, it frequently responds positively to gentle herbal treatments.

Echinacea Spray

Makes about I cup

Echinacea effectively combats candida, a common culprit in severe cases of dandruff, while witch hazel provides relief from the persistent itching. If your scalp is damaged from itching, the witch hazel will help it heal. This spray can remain fresh for up to a year when stored in the refrigerator.

Ingredients

I cup witch hazel

2 tablespoons echinacea tincture

Steps

Combine the ingredients in a sleek glass bottle with a spray top.

Gently shake to blend thoroughly.

Apply I or 2 spritzes to each part of your scalp where you're experiencing dandruff.

Gently apply the spray using your fingertips, followed by brushing or combing your hair. You have the option to style your hair as you normally would and keep the spray in throughout the day if you prefer, or you can choose to leave it in for I to 2 hours and then wash it out with shampoo. For optimal results, use on a daily basis.

Precautions: Avoid using echinacea if you have an autoimmune disorder or if you are allergic to ragweed.

Rosemary Conditioner

Makes I cup

This straightforward antifungal remedy combines a natural, unscented conditioner tailored to your specific hair type with rosemary essential oil, which is highly concentrated and delightfully fragrant. If you don't happen to have rosemary essential oil on hand, you can easily substitute it with tincture.

Ingredients

I cup natural, unscented herbal conditioner like Stonybrook Botanicals

40 drops rosemary essential oil

Steps

Combine the conditioner and essential oil in a large bowl, ensuring they are thoroughly blended using a whisk or fork. Transfer it to a BPA-free plastic bottle with a squeeze top using a funnel.

After shampooing, apply a dollop of conditioner to your scalp, adjusting the amount as necessary to ensure full coverage. Wait for 2 to 5 minutes, then rinse the conditioner out with cool water. Style your hair as you normally would. For optimal results, use on a daily basis.

Diaper Rash

Diaper rash can sometimes occur, even if you are careful about changing your baby's diaper. It can cause pain, redness, and swelling. Herbal remedies are perfect for your baby's delicate skin, as they are free from any harmful talc or petroleum products commonly found in commercial preparations.

Chamomile-Echinacea Gel

Makes about ½ cup

Aloe, chamomile, and echinacea combine to provide gentle relief for your child's rash. Echinacea specifically targets yeast, a common fungus that can exacerbate diaper rash. This gel can maintain its freshness for a duration of 2 weeks when stored in the refrigerator.

Ingredients

I tablespoon dried chamomile

I tablespoon chopped dried echinacea root

½ cup water

¼ cup aloe vera gel

Steps

Combine the chamomile and echinacea with the water in a saucepan. Bring the mixture to a boil over high heat, then lower the heat to a gentle simmer. Cook the mixture until it is reduced by half, then take it off the heat and let it cool completely.

Moisten a piece of cheesecloth and place it over the opening of a funnel. Transfer the mixture through the funnel into a glass bowl. Squeeze the cheesecloth until all the liquid has been extracted.

Combine the aloe vera gel with the liquid and mix it together using a whisk. Place the completed gel into a sterilized glass jar. Make sure to seal the jar securely and keep it in the refrigerator.

After every diaper change, gently apply a thin layer to the affected areas using a cotton cosmetic pad. Ensure the gel is fully absorbed before applying the Comfrey-Thyme Salve and re-diapering. Make sure to continue using this gel for at least 3 days after the diaper rash has cleared up.

Precautions: Do not use echinacea if your baby has an autoimmune disorder.

Comfrey-Thyme Salve

Makes about I cup

Comfrey is known for its healing properties, while thyme has strong antibacterial effects. This luxurious salve also offers a protective shield against moisture, allowing your baby's delicate skin to heal. It might be a good idea to make a double batch and have one jar in the diaper bag and another near your home changing area. This salve has a long shelf life of one year when stored in a cool, dark place.

Ingredients

I cup light olive oil

I ounce dried comfrey

I ounce dried thyme

I ounce beeswax

Steps

Combine the olive oil, comfrey, and thyme in a slow cooker. Choose the lowest heat setting, cover the slow cooker, and let the herbs steep in the oil for 3 to 5 hours. Switch off the heat and let the infused oil cool down.

Heat a small amount of water in the base of a double boiler until it simmers.

Lower the heat to a low setting.

Place a cheesecloth over the top portion of the double boiler. Add the infused oil and squeeze the cheesecloth tightly to extract all the oil.

Dispose of the cheesecloth and used herbs.

Combine the beeswax with the infused oil and carefully position the double boiler on the base.

Warm slowly over low heat. Once the beeswax has completely melted, carefully take the pan off the heat. Efficiently transfer the salve into pristine, dry jars or tins and let it cool entirely before sealing.

After each diaper change, gently apply a thin layer to your baby's diaper area using your fingers or a gauze pad. Begin with a small amount of salve, adjusting as necessary.

Dry Skin

Factors such as dehydration, indoor air temperature, and prolonged hot showers can all contribute to dry skin. Regular moisturizing can be beneficial, along with the use of humidifiers and treatments that incorporate calming herbs.

Chickweed-Aloe Gel

Makes about ½ cup

Chickweed and aloe vera work together to nourish and hydrate the skin. This gel is designed to absorb quickly and leave no odor behind. When kept in a cool environment, it will remain fresh for a duration of 2 weeks.

Ingredients

½ cup water

¼ cup dried chickweed

¼ cup aloe vera gel

Steps

Combine the water and chickweed in a saucepan. Bring the mixture to a rapid boil over high heat, then gently lower the heat to a simmer. Cook the mixture until it reduces by half, then take it off the heat and let it cool completely.

Moisten a piece of cheesecloth and carefully place it over the opening of a funnel. Pour the mixture through the funnel into a high-quality glass bowl. Extract the liquid from the herbs by firmly squeezing the cheesecloth until all the liquid has been released.

Combine the aloe vera gel with the liquid and mix it together using a whisk. Transfer the finished gel to a clean squeeze bottle that is free from BPA. Make sure to seal it securely and place it in the refrigerator.

Apply a thin layer to all affected areas twice per day using your fingertips.

Begin with a small amount and adjust the quantity for future use based on the dryness of your skin.

Calendula-Comfrey Body Butter

Makes about 2½ cups

Calendula and comfrey have soothing properties that can help heal irritated skin, while the emollients in this product help to keep your skin moisturized. Feel free to add your preferred essential oils to give it a delightful fragrance. When properly stored, it can maintain its freshness for up to a year.

Ingredients

½ cup cocoa butter

½ cup coconut oil

½ cup jojoba oil

½ cup shea butter

2 ounces dried calendula

2 ounces dried comfrey

Steps

Combine all the ingredients in a slow cooker. Choose the lowest heat setting, cover the slow cooker, and let the herbs steep for 3 to 5 hours. Switch off the heat and let the infused oil cool down.

Place a piece of cheesecloth gently over a large mixing bowl. Add the infused oil and squeeze the cheesecloth tightly until all the oil has been extracted.

Get rid of the cheesecloth and the herbs that have been used.

Put the bowl in the refrigerator and allow the mixture to cool for approximately an hour, or until it starts to firm up.

Using a hand mixer or immersion blender, whip the body butter for 10 minutes, or until it becomes light and fluffy. Place the bowl back in the refrigerator for 15 minutes, and then carefully transfer the body butter into clean, dry jars with secure lids.

Apply a small amount to dry skin using your fingers. Adjust the amount as desired and apply daily for smooth and luxurious skin.

Earache

An earache occurs when the sensory nerve endings in the eardrum react to pressure. Consider using herbal remedies at the first indication of discomfort. If the pain worsens or persists, it is important to consult with a medical professional. Severe ear infections have the potential to spread or result in permanent hearing impairment.

Blue Vervain Infusion and Poultice

Makes 1 treatment

Blue vervain is known for its pain-relieving properties and ability to improve circulation. This treatment has a dual effect. The warm poultice provides soothing relief to the ear area externally, while the infusion, when consumed, helps alleviate the discomfort in the throat that often accompanies an earache. The infusion has a bitter taste, so you might consider adding a sweetener to help conceal it.

Ingredients

2 teaspoons dried blue vervain

1 cup boiling water

Steps

Place the blue vervain in a tea infuser and gently immerse it in a mug. Pour the boiling water over it.

Let the infusion steep for 10 minutes.

Take out the infuser from the water and let it cool down until it's hot but not too hot to touch. Move the blue vervain to a piece of cheesecloth and neatly fold the cloth into a 4-inch square.

Apply the poultice gently to your ear and enjoy the tea at a leisurely pace. To reactivate the poultice for a second use, simply wrap it in a moist towel and heat it in the microwave for 5 to 10 seconds.

Continue the treatment up to three times per day until your earache subsides.

Garlic-Mullein Infused Oil

Makes 2 tablespoons

Garlic and mullein flowers have powerful antibacterial and anti-inflammatory properties that can effectively alleviate an earache in no time. This oil has a long shelf life of up to a year when stored in a cool, dark place.

Ingredients

2 tablespoons light olive oil

2 teaspoons crushed or finely chopped dried or freeze-dried garlic

2 teaspoons dried mullein flowers

Steps

Bring a small amount of water to a gentle simmer in the base of a double boiler.

Lower the heat to a lower setting.

Combine the olive oil, garlic, and mullein flowers in a glass measuring cup.

Position the measuring cup in the top section of the double boiler and let the herbs infuse in the oil for a duration of 3 to 5 hours. Switch off the heat and let the infused oil cool down.

Place a piece of cheesecloth gently over a small bowl. Add the infused oil and wring and twist the cheesecloth until all the oil has been extracted. Remove the cheesecloth and used herbs.

Transfer the infused oil into a dry, sterilized bottle with a dropper top and wait for it to cool completely before sealing it.

Using the dropper top, carefully apply 2 to 3 drops into the ear. Insert a cotton ball into the ear and allow it to remain there for 15 minutes. Continue this routine two or three times daily until the earache subsides.

Precautions: Garlic may cause a skin rash in sensitive individuals; discontinue if irritation occurs.

Eczema

Commonly referred to as atopic dermatitis, eczema is identified by irritated patches of thick, red, scaly skin that can cause intense itching. This allergic skin condition has a tendency to come and go, often coinciding with seasonal or dietary allergy symptoms.

Calendula-Goldenseal Spray

Makes I cup

Calendula and goldenseal provide antiseptic and anti-inflammatory benefits, while witch hazel helps to soothe redness, itching, and scaling. This spray will remain fresh for up to a year if stored in a cool, dark place.

Ingredients

I ounce dried calendula

I ounce dried goldenseal root

¼ cup jojoba oil

¾ cup witch hazel

Steps

Combine the calendula, goldenseal, and jojoba oil in a slow cooker. Choose the lowest heat setting, cover the slow cooker, and let the herbs steep in the oil for 3 to 5 hours. Switch off the heat and let the infused oil cool down.

Place a piece of cheesecloth gently over a bowl. Add the infused oil and squeeze the cheesecloth until all the oil is extracted. Dispose of the used herbs.

Mix the infused oil and witch hazel in a glass bottle with a spray top, preferably dark-colored. Handle with care.

Apply I or 2 spritzes to the affected area. Gently apply the spray and let it soak in. Continue this routine two or three times per day until the eczema fades.

Comfrey Salve

Makes about I cup

Comfrey is known for its ability to calm and relieve irritated, itchy skin. It additionally aids in smoothing rough areas and preventing cracking. Comfrey is known for its ability to stimulate cell regeneration, which can accelerate the healing process and potentially aid in repairing damage caused by eczema. This salve can maintain its effectiveness for up to a year if stored in a cool, dark place.

Ingredients

2 ounces dried comfrey

I cup light olive oil

I ounce beeswax

20 drops vitamin E oil

Steps

Combine the comfrey and olive oil in a slow cooker. Choose the lowest heat setting, cover the slow cooker, and let the herbs steep in the oil for 3 to 5 hours. Disable the heat and let the infused oil cool down.

Heat up a small amount of water in the base of a double boiler until it simmers.

Lower the heat to a low setting.

Place a piece of cheesecloth over the top of the double boiler. Add the infused oil, squeezing the cheesecloth until all the oil has been extracted.

Dispose of the cheesecloth and used herbs.

Combine the beeswax with the infused oil and carefully position the double boiler on the base.

Warm slowly over low heat. Once the beeswax has completely melted, carefully remove the pan from the heat source. After letting the blend cool down a bit, simply incorporate the vitamin E oil using a whisk. Efficiently transfer the salve into pristine, dry jars or tins and let it cool entirely before sealing.

Apply a small amount to areas of eczema, adjusting the quantity as necessary. Continue this routine two or three times per day until the eczema gradually fades away.

Fever

Allow your body to naturally combat infection by embracing the power of fever. If your fever worsens or persists, febrifuge herbs can be beneficial in reducing it. It is crucial to be extremely cautious and proactive in seeking medical assistance if your child has a fever. For infants under 4 months old, it is crucial to seek immediate medical attention if their body temperature reaches 100.4°F or higher. Older children should be seen promptly for a fever of 104°F or higher.

Feverfew Syrup

Makes about 2 cups

Feverfew is known for its ability to effectively reduce fevers. This syrup is perfect for children as it is gentle and easy to take. Plus, it can stay fresh for up to 6 months when refrigerated.

Ingredients

2 ounces dried feverfew

2 cups water

1 cup honey

Steps

Combine the feverfew and water in a saucepan. Simmer the liquid over low heat, partially covering it with a lid, until it is reduced by half.

Pour the contents of the saucepan into a glass measuring cup, then strain the mixture through a dampened piece of cheesecloth back into the saucepan, squeezing out the liquid from the cheesecloth.

Include the honey and gently heat the mixture on low, stirring continuously until it reaches a temperature of 105°F to 110°F.

Transfer the syrup to a sterilized jar or bottle and keep it in the refrigerator.

Take 1 tablespoon by mouth three times daily until your symptoms improve.

For optimal results, it is recommended that children under the age of 12 take 1 teaspoon three times per day.

Blue Vervain–Raspberry Leaf Tincture

Makes about 2 cups

Blue vervain and raspberry leaf are highly effective in reducing fever in a gentle manner. This tincture will stay fresh for up to 6 years if stored in a cool, dark place.

Ingredients

4 ounces dried blue vervain

4 ounces dried raspberry leaf

2 cups unflavored 80-proof vodka

Steps

Combine the herbs in a sterilized pint jar. Pour the vodka into the jar, ensuring it reaches the brim and fully submerges the herbs.

Make sure to secure the jar firmly and give it a good shake. Keep it in a cool, dark cabinet and give it a good shake every week for 6 to 8 weeks. If any of the alcohol evaporates, simply add more vodka to fill the jar to the top once again.

Moisten a piece of cheesecloth and carefully place it over the opening of a funnel. Transfer the tincture through the funnel into a clean pint jar. Extract the liquid from the herbs by firmly squeezing the cheesecloth until all the liquid has been released. Remove the roots and carefully transfer the completed tincture into glass bottles of a dark color.

Administer 10 drops orally two or three times per day. If the flavor is too intense for your liking, you have the option to dilute it by mixing it with a glass of water or juice and consuming it.

Flu

Influenza, caused by a virus that mutates frequently, often presents symptoms similar to the common cold. Getting a yearly flu shot is highly recommended, particularly if you are regularly exposed to sick individuals or belong to a high-risk group. If you happen to come down with the flu, herbs can be beneficial in alleviating your symptoms and expediting your recovery.

Catnip-Hyssop Tea

Makes I cup

Both catnip and hyssop have anti-inflammatory properties that can help alleviate symptoms such as a sore throat and body ache. Additionally, they can enhance your immune system, helping to combat the flu virus. This tea is incredibly soothing and perfect for enjoying before a nap or bedtime.

Ingredients

I cup boiling water

I teaspoon dried catnip

I teaspoon dried hyssop

Steps

Transfer the hot water into a spacious mug. Include the dried herbs, place a lid on the mug, and let the tea steep for I0 minutes.

Take your time and savor the tea as you enjoy the soothing steam. Can be repeated up to four times daily.

Precautions: Do not use hyssop or catnip during pregnancy. Omit the hyssop if you have epilepsy

Garlic, Echinacea, and Goldenseal Syrup

Makes 2 cups

Garlic, echinacea, and goldenseal are powerful antiviral herbs that can support your body's natural defense against the flu. This syrup has a strong flavor despite the honey; you might find it more enjoyable if you consume it with a teaspoon of lemon juice. When stored in a cool environment, it can maintain its freshness for up to 6 months.

Ingredients

I ounce dried or freeze-dried garlic, chopped

I ounce dried echinacea root, chopped

I ounce dried goldenseal root, chopped

2 cups water

I cup honey

Steps

Combine the herbs and water in a saucepan. Heat the liquid gently until it simmers. Cover it partially with a lid and let the liquid reduce by half.

Pour the contents of the saucepan into a glass measuring cup. Then, strain the mixture back into the saucepan using a dampened piece of cheesecloth. Squeeze the cheesecloth until no more liquid is extracted.

Include the honey and gently heat the mixture on a low flame, stirring continuously and ceasing when the temperature reaches 105°F to 110°F.

Transfer the syrup to a sterilized jar or bottle and keep it chilled in the refrigerator.

Take 1 tablespoon by mouth three times daily until your symptoms improve.

For optimal results, it is recommended that children under the age of 12 take 1 teaspoon three times per day.

Precautions: Do not use echinacea if you are allergic to ragweed or have an autoimmune disease.

Gingivitis

Even with regular brushing, gingivitis can still develop. This dental condition often leads to gum recession and, over time, can cause teeth to become loose. Make flossing a regular part of your routine and schedule biannual dental cleanings. Using herbs can contribute to maintaining the health of your teeth and gums in addition to regular professional cleanings.

Calendula-Chamomile Mouth Rinse

Makes 2 cups

Calendula and chamomile work together to soothe inflammation and combat infections. This mouth rinse has a delightful floral flavor and provides relief to sore gums, promoting the healing of damaged tissue. This rinse can stay fresh for up to a week if stored in the refrigerator.

Ingredients

I ounce dried calendula

I ounce dried chamomile

4 cups water

Steps

Combine the herbs and water in a saucepan. Slowly heat the liquid until it simmers, then partially cover it with a lid and let it reduce by half.

Pour the contents of the saucepan into a glass measuring cup. Next, strain the mixture back into the saucepan using a dampened piece of cheesecloth. Squeeze the cheesecloth to remove any remaining liquid.

Transfer the mouth rinse to a clean jar or bottle and store it in a cool place.

Use 2 tablespoons twice a day until your symptoms improve. Remember to spit the rinse into the sink instead of swallowing it. For children under age 12, it is recommended to take 1 tablespoon twice per day.

Goldenseal-Sage Oil Pull

Makes 24 treatments

This recipe combines goldenseal, sage, and coconut oil to create a potent treatment that aids in reducing inflammation and promoting the healing of sore gums. If you are new to oil pulling, it's best to start slowly and gradually increase the duration of your treatment.
This blend will remain fresh for up to 6 months if stored in a cool, dark place.

Ingredients

1 ounce dried goldenseal root, chopped

1 ounce dried sage, crumbled

½ cup coconut oil

Steps

Combine the herbs and coconut oil in a slow cooker. Choose the lowest heat setting, cover the slow cooker, and let the herbs steep in the oil for 3 to 5 hours. Disable the heat and let the infused oil cool down.

Place a piece of cheesecloth gently over a bowl. Add the infused oil and squeeze the cheesecloth tightly until all the oil is extracted. Remove the cheesecloth and used herbs.

Transfer the infused coconut oil to a clean, dry jar and let it cool completely before sealing it.

Use I teaspoon of the oil pulling solution and let it dissolve in your mouth. Gently move it around and between your teeth, but avoid swallowing. Hold the solution in your mouth for a maximum of 15 minutes, adjusting the amount as necessary.

After completing the task, dispose of the used oil by spitting it into a paper towel and throwing it away in the trash. Please avoid pouring oil down the sink as it can cause plumbing issues.

Hair Loss

Although hair loss is commonly associated with men, women can also experience this condition. Thinning hair can be caused by a variety of factors, including overstyling, stress, and imbalances in vitamins.

Herbs are generally not effective for genetic hair loss, but they can promote hair growth in various other cases.

Ginger Scalp Treatment

Makes ½ cup

Ginger enhances blood flow to the scalp, promoting the activation of hair follicles. This treatment will remain fresh for up to 2 months when stored in the refrigerator.

Ingredients

2 ounces fresh gingerroot, chopped

¼ cup sesame oil

Steps

Combine the ginger and sesame oil in a slow cooker. Choose the lowest heat setting, cover the slow cooker, and let the herbs steep in the oil for 3 to 5 hours. Disable the heat and let the infused oil cool down.

Place a piece of cheesecloth gently over a bowl. Add the infused oil and squeeze the cheesecloth until all the oil has been extracted. Dispose of the used ginger.

Transfer the sesame oil to a clean, dry bottle or jar and let it cool completely before sealing.

Before shampooing your hair, apply 1 tablespoon to the scalp. Apply it gently.

Keep the treatment on for 30 minutes, then wash and condition your hair as you normally would. Make sure to repeat three to four times per week.

Precautions: Do not use ginger if you take prescription blood thinners, have gallbladder disease, or have a bleeding disorder.

Ginkgo-Rosemary Tonic

Makes about 1 cup

Ginkgo and rosemary, along with witch hazel, work together to enhance circulation in the scalp, providing a boost to your hair follicles. Rosemary enhances the luster and resilience of your hair, contributing to an enhanced appearance and boosted self-confidence. This tonic will remain fresh for up to 6 months when stored in the refrigerator.

Ingredients

½ ounce dried ginkgo biloba

½ ounce dried rosemary leaves

2 tablespoons fractionated coconut oil

1 cup witch hazel

Steps

Combine the herbs and fractionated coconut oil in a slow cooker. Choose the lowest heat setting, cover the slow cooker, and let the herbs steep in the oil for 3 to 5 hours. Disable the heat and let the infused oil cool down.

Place a piece of cheesecloth gently over a bowl. Add the infused oil and squeeze the cheesecloth tightly until all the oil is extracted. Remove the cheesecloth and used herbs.

Mix the witch hazel with the infused oil in a glass bottle with a spray top. Shake gently to ensure thorough blending.

After washing and conditioning your hair, simply apply a light mist of 1 or 2 spritzes to areas where hair loss is a concern, adjusting the amount as necessary.

Gently massage the scalp using your fingertips. Make sure to repeat once or twice per day.

Precautions: Do not use ginkgo biloba if you are taking a monoamine oxidase inhibitor (MAOI) for depression. Ginkgo biloba enhances the effect of blood thinners; talk to your doctor before use. Do not use rosemary if you have epilepsy.

Halitosis

Unpleasant and embarrassing, bad breath can be quite bothersome. Fortunately, it's also quite simple to address. Begin by ensuring you stay properly hydrated, as a lack of moisture in the mouth can create an ideal breeding ground for bacteria. Make sure to maintain good oral hygiene by being extra diligent with brushing and flossing. If herbs are not effective, it is advisable to consult with your doctor. Persistent bad breath can be a sign of an underlying medical issue.

Peppermint-Sage Mouthwash

Makes about 2 cups

Peppermint and sage work together to keep your breath fresh, while the powerful formula in this mouthwash effectively eliminates germs. When prepared with vodka and stored in a cool, dark place, the rinse can maintain its freshness for a remarkable 6 years.

Ingredients

6 ounces dried peppermint

2 ounces dried sage

2 cups unflavored 80-proof vodka

Steps

Combine the herbs in a sterilized pint jar. Fill the jar to the brim with vodka, ensuring that the herbs are completely covered.

Make sure to securely seal the jar and give it a good shake. Keep it in a cool, dark cabinet and give it a good shake every few days for 6 to 8 weeks. If any of the alcohol evaporates, simply add more vodka to fill the jar.

Moisten a piece of cheesecloth and carefully place it over the opening of a funnel. Transfer the tincture through the funnel into a clean pint jar. Squeeze out the liquid from the herbs. Dispose of the used herbs and pour the completed tincture into glass bottles of a dark color.

After brushing your teeth, rinse with 1 tablespoon of mouthwash. Make sure to repeat at least twice per day, and feel free to do it more frequently if you prefer.

Ginger-Mint Gunpowder Green Tea

Makes about 30 servings.

When lemon and spearmint are combined with gunpowder green tea, the polyphenols present in the tea act as antioxidants. These antioxidants have the ability to eliminate certain compounds that are linked to issues like bad breath, tooth decay, and even mouth cancer.

Ingredients

2 lemons

1 (4-inch) piece gingerroot

2 bunches spearmint

1 cup gunpowder green tea leaves

1 cup boiling water

Steps

Prepare the lemons by peeling them, removing the pith, and cutting the rinds into thin slivers.

Put the rinds on a metal rack. (You can save the juiced lemons for another purpose.)

Peel the gingerroot and slice it into thin pieces. Arrange them on the rack along with the lemon rinds.

Take off the leaves from the spearmint stems, making sure to keep the leaves whole. Remove the stems and arrange the spearmint leaves on the rack alongside the lemon rinds and gingerroot.

Allow the lemon rinds, gingerroot, and spearmint leaves to dry naturally at room temperature until they are completely dry and brittle, which usually takes around 24 hours. Ensure that all moisture has been completely eliminated. Break up the spearmint leaves into small fragments.

Combine the lemon rinds, ginger, spearmint leaves, and tea leaves in a spacious bowl. Once the ingredients are fully combined, carefully transfer the mixture into a tightly sealed container. Keep at a moderate temperature for a month.

To prepare the tea, carefully pour the hot water into a spacious mug. Add 2 teaspoons of the tea mixture, cover the mug, and let the tea steep for 10 minutes.

Enjoy a cup of tea.

Hangover

Indulging a bit too much is common, but there's no need to suffer through the consequences in total discomfort. Explore solutions that target your specific issues such as headache, nausea, and fatigue, while also incorporating remedies that aid in the detoxification process.

Feverfew-Hops Tea

Makes I cup

Feverfew can effectively address your headache, while hops have a calming effect to help you relax. This tea has a powerful effect that can assist you in falling asleep, allowing your body to recuperate more quickly.

Ingredients

I cup boiling water

I teaspoon dried feverfew

I teaspoon dried hops

Steps

Transfer the hot water into a spacious mug. Include the dried herbs, place a lid on the mug, and let the tea steep for 10 minutes.

Take your time and savor the tea. Can be repeated up to three times per day.

Milk Thistle Tincture

Makes about 2 cups

Milk thistle is beneficial for the liver as it aids in the detoxification process. This solution may not provide instant relief, but it can help alleviate some strain on your system. When stored in an optimal environment, the product can maintain its freshness for an extended period of time.

Ingredients

8 ounces dried milk thistle

2 cups unflavored 80-proof vodka

Steps

Place the milk thistle in a sanitized pint jar. Fill the jar to the brim with vodka, ensuring that the herbs are completely submerged.

Make sure to secure the jar firmly and give it a good shake. Keep it in a cool, dark cabinet and give it a good shake every week for 6 to 8 weeks. If any of the alcohol evaporates, simply add more vodka to fill the jar to the top once again.

Moisten a piece of cheesecloth and carefully place it over the opening of a funnel. Transfer the tincture through the funnel into a clean, sterilized pint jar. Extract the liquid from the herbs by firmly squeezing the cheesecloth until all the liquid has been released. Dispose of the used herbs and pour the completed tincture into glass bottles with a dark color.

Take 10 drops orally two or three times per day for 7 to 10 days after excessive consumption. If the flavor is too intense for your liking, you have the option to dilute it by mixing it with water or juice before consumption. If you prefer not to consume alcohol, you can incorporate the tincture into a cup of tea prepared with boiling water. The alcohol will evaporate in approximately 5 minutes.

Headache

Headaches can be triggered by various factors such as stress, muscle tension, caffeine withdrawal, eyestrain, and high blood pressure. If you experience frequent or persistent headaches, it is advisable to consult with a medical professional, as they may be indicative of an underlying health condition.

Blue Vervain–Catnip Tea

Makes 1 cup

Blue vervain and catnip work in harmony to enhance circulation and induce a sense of calm, while also providing relief from tension. This blend is perfect for relieving stress headaches.

Ingredients

1 cup boiling water

1 teaspoon dried blue vervain

1 teaspoon dried catnip

Steps

Transfer the hot water into a spacious mug. Include the dried herbs, place a lid on the mug, and let the tea steep for 10 minutes.

Take your time and savor the tea. Feel free to repeat this up to three times per day.

Skullcap Tincture

Makes about 2 cups

Skullcap is a gentle sedative that can provide relief for nerve pain. If you experience migraines and are unable to use feverfew, skullcap may be a viable alternative to explore.

This tincture offers fast relief. If you would prefer a more convenient option, skullcap is also available in capsule form. When stored in an optimal environment, this tincture can maintain its freshness for an impressive duration of 6 years.

Ingredients

8 ounces skullcap

2 cups unflavored 80-proof vodka

Steps

Place the skullcap in a sanitized pint jar. Fill the jar to the brim with vodka, ensuring that the herbs are completely submerged.

Make sure to securely seal the jar and give it a good shake. Keep it in a cool, dark cabinet and give it a good shake every few days for 6 to 8 weeks. If any of the alcohol evaporates, make sure to replenish it with more vodka until the jar is completely filled again.

Moisten a piece of cheesecloth and carefully place it over the opening of a funnel. Transfer the tincture through the funnel into a clean pint jar. Extract the liquid from the herbs by firmly squeezing the cheesecloth until all the liquid has been released. Dispose of the used herbs and pour the completed tincture into glass bottles of a dark color.

For headache relief, simply take I teaspoon orally two or three times per day. If the flavor is too intense for your liking, you have the option to dilute it by mixing it with water or juice before consumption.

Heartburn

The intense discomfort caused by heartburn is a common symptom of gastroesophageal reflux disease (GERD), a digestive disorder that occurs when stomach acid flows into the esophagus. GERD can be triggered by various factors such as excessive acid production, obesity, overeating, wearing tight clothing, and several other factors. If you are pregnant, heartburn may occur due to the increased pressure on your stomach caused by your growing baby. Herbs can provide relief for heartburn, offering a temporary solution as you investigate the root cause.

Fresh Ginger Tea

Makes I cup

Ginger enhances blood circulation throughout the body and can expedite recovery from heartburn. The soothing properties of this product help alleviate the irritation in your esophagus caused by stomach acid.

Ingredients

I cup boiling water

I tablespoon chopped fresh gingerroot

Steps

Transfer the hot water into a spacious mug. Include the ginger, place a lid on the mug, and let the tea steep for 10 minutes.

Take your time and savor the tea as you enjoy the soothing steam. Use up to four times per day as needed for heartburn relief.

Fennel-Angelica Syrup

Makes 2 cups

Fennel and angelica enhance blood circulation in the digestive system and provide a soothing effect to an irritated esophagus, promoting faster digestion. This syrup has a long shelf life of 6 months when stored in the refrigerator.

Ingredients

1 ounce dried angelica

1 tablespoon fennel seeds

2 cups water

1 cup honey

Steps

Combine the herbs and water in a saucepan. Simmer the liquid gently over low heat, covering it partially with a lid, until it is reduced by half.

Pour the contents of the saucepan into a glass measuring cup. Then, strain the mixture back into the saucepan using a dampened piece of cheesecloth, squeezing out all the liquid.

Incorporate the honey and gently heat the mixture on a low flame, ensuring to stir continuously until the temperature reaches 105°F to 110°F.

Transfer the syrup to a sterilized jar or bottle and keep it in the refrigerator.

Take 1 tablespoon by mouth three times daily until your heartburn symptoms improve.

High Blood Pressure

If left untreated, high blood pressure, also known as hypertension, can significantly raise the risk of early cognitive decline, heart disease, kidney failure, and stroke. Incorporating healthy habits like weight loss, exercise, and meditation can naturally promote healing. If you are unable to lower your blood pressure within 2 months, it is important to seek immediate medical attention from your doctor.

Angelica Infusion

Makes 1 quart

Angelica contains compounds that have similar effects to calcium channel blockers, which are commonly prescribed to lower high blood pressure by relaxing and widening blood vessels. This infusion has a slightly bitter taste, but you can easily enhance its flavor by adding a touch of sweetener or juice to your liking. When stored in a cool environment, it will remain fresh for 3 days.

Ingredients

4 teaspoons dried angelica

4 cups boiling water

4 teaspoons fresh lemon juice

Steps

Combine the dried angelica and boiling water in a teapot. Make sure to cover the pot and let the infusion steep for 10 minutes before adding the lemon juice.

Take your time and savor a cup of the infusion. You have the option to refrigerate the remaining portion and enjoy it gradually over the next few days, whether you prefer to reheat it or have it over ice.

Dandelion-Lavender Tincture

Makes about 2 cups

Dandelions are a great natural way to regulate salt levels and reduce blood pressure. The scent and oils of lavender have a calming effect on the nervous system, promoting relaxation and balance.

Ingredients

4 ounces dried dandelion root, finely chopped

4 ounces dried lavender leaves, chopped

2 cups unflavored 80-proof vodka

Steps

Combine the herbs in a sterilized pint jar. Pour the vodka into the jar, ensuring it reaches the brim and fully submerges the herbs.

Make sure to seal the jar securely and give it a good shake. Keep it in a cool, dark cabinet and give it a good shake every few days for 6 to 8 weeks. If any of the alcohol evaporates, make sure to replenish it with more vodka until the jar is once again filled to the brim.

Moisten a piece of cheesecloth and carefully place it over the opening of a funnel. Transfer the tincture through the funnel into a clean pint jar. Extract the liquid from the herbs by firmly squeezing the cheesecloth until all the liquid has been released. Dispose of the used herbs and pour the completed tincture into glass bottles of a dark color.

Administer 10 drops orally two or three times per day. If the flavor is too intense for your liking, you have the option to dilute it by mixing it with a glass of water or juice before consumption. Keep up with your efforts to make lifestyle changes and take positive steps to enhance your blood pressure.

Precautions: It is advised to avoid using this tincture for more than 2 months. Using dandelions excessively may result in a significant decrease in blood pressure levels, which can be potentially dangerous. When consumed orally, excessive amounts of lavender may cause constipation, headaches, and an increase in appetite. If you encounter any negative side effects, it is important to seek immediate medical advice from your physician.

Indigestion

Feeling bloated, experiencing belching, and feeling uncomfortable are indications that you may have consumed something that didn't sit well with your stomach, or that you may have indulged a little too much in a beloved dish. Herbs provide fast relief without any of the potential side effects that may come with commercial antacids.

Chamomile-Angelica Tea

Makes 1 cup

Angelica and chamomile have a soothing effect on the muscles in the gastrointestinal tract, promoting better circulation and maintaining a healthy flow. Adding a teaspoon of honey and a squeeze of fresh lemon can enhance the taste of your tea.

Ingredients

1 cup boiling water

1 teaspoon dried angelica

1 teaspoon dried chamomile

Steps

Transfer the hot water into a spacious mug. Include the dried herbs, cover the mug, and let the tea steep for 10 minutes.

Take your time and savor the tea. Repeat up to four times daily.

Ginger Syrup

Makes 2 cups

Ginger has a calming effect on the digestive tract and promotes better blood circulation, which can aid in digestion. For even faster relief, try taking this remedy with a teaspoon of fresh lemon juice. This syrup can be stored in the refrigerator for up to 6 months while maintaining its freshness.

Ingredients

2 ounces fresh gingerroot, chopped

2 cups water

1 cup honey

Steps

Combine the ginger and water in a saucepan. Heat the liquid gently until it simmers. Cover it partially with a lid and let the liquid reduce by half.

Pour the contents of the saucepan into a glass measuring cup, and then strain the mixture back into the saucepan using a dampened piece of cheesecloth. Squeeze the cheesecloth to remove any remaining liquid.

Incorporate the honey and gently heat the mixture on a low flame, ensuring to stir continuously until the temperature reaches 105°F to 110°F.

Transfer the syrup to a sterilized jar or bottle and keep it in the refrigerator.

Take 1 tablespoon orally three or four times per day until your symptoms improve. For children under age 12, it is recommended to take 1 teaspoon up to three times per day.

Insect Bites

Mosquitos, chiggers, biting gnats, and fleas are among the pests that can leave irritating, itchy bites on your skin. Occasionally, these bothersome bites can cause discomfort, making it difficult to concentrate or get a good night's rest. Fortunately, there are natural remedies available to provide relief.

Fresh Basil-Mullein Salve

Makes I treatment

Basil and mullein provide anti-inflammatory benefits, and basil also contains eugenol, a constituent known for its itch-numbing properties. This remedy utilizes the natural properties of honey to effectively bind the herbs to your skin, promoting faster healing of your bug bites. If you have a large number of insect bites or if your entire family is affected, you can easily increase the recipe to ensure there is enough for everyone. When stored in the refrigerator, it remains fresh for up to 2 days.

Ingredients

I tablespoon fresh basil

I tablespoon fresh mullein

I tablespoon raw honey

Steps

Combine all the ingredients in a mini food processor. Blend the ingredients until they form a smooth paste.

Using your fingertip or a cotton swab, gently apply a small amount of the blend to each of your insect bites.

Store any remaining salve in a small container with a secure lid and keep it refrigerated for future use. Continue the treatment whenever itching resurfaces.

Peppermint-Plantain Balm

Makes about 5 tablespoons (enough to fill 5 lip balm tubes)

If you frequently encounter buggy environments, you'll appreciate the convenience and user-friendly nature of these tubes of insect bite balm. The peppermint and plantain provide soothing relief and promote faster healing for your skin. Additionally, this balm can be used to keep your lips feeling soft and smooth. This remedy has a long shelf life of up to a year when stored in a cool, dark place.

Ingredients

1 tablespoon dried peppermint

1 tablespoon dried plantain

2 tablespoons jojoba oil

1 tablespoon light olive oil

1 tablespoon cocoa butter

4 teaspoons grated beeswax or beeswax pastilles

3 drops vitamin E oil

20 drops peppermint essential oil (optional)

Steps

Combine the herbs with the jojoba oil, olive oil, and cocoa butter in a slow cooker. Choose the lowest heat setting, cover the slow cooker, and let the herbs steep in the oil for 3 to 5 hours. Switch off the heat and let the infused oil cool down.

Heat a small amount of water in the base of a double boiler until it simmers.

Lower the heat to a low setting.

Place a piece of cheesecloth over the top section of the double boiler. Add the infused oil, then squeeze and twist the cheesecloth until all the oil has been extracted. Dispose of the cheesecloth and used herbs.

Combine the beeswax with the infused oil and carefully position the double boiler on the base.

Take the pan off the heat once the wax has melted, and then include the vitamin E oil and peppermint essential oil (if desired). Pour the mixture into clean, dry lip balm tubes or tins and let it cool completely before capping.

Apply a small amount of balm to each insect bite as often as necessary to alleviate itching.

Laryngitis

When your voice box becomes swollen and inflamed from infection, irritation, or overuse, laryngitis occurs. If the problem persists, it is advisable to consult a doctor as prolonged hoarseness may indicate an underlying illness. While herbs can provide some relief, professional medical attention is recommended.

Mullein-Sage Tea

Makes I cup

Mullein and sage can provide relief and promote healing for laryngitis symptoms and irritated tissue. This calming solution possesses a potent herbal flavor; you might consider incorporating a teaspoon of lemon juice or honey to enhance its palatability.

Ingredients

I cup boiling water

I teaspoon dried mullein

I teaspoon dried sage

Steps

Transfer the hot water into a spacious mug. Include the dried herbs, cover the mug, and let the tea steep for 10 minutes.

Indulge in a moment of pure relaxation as you savor your favorite tea. Feel free to repeat as often as needed.

Ginger Gargle

Makes I cup

This recipe includes ginger, which can help alleviate pain and reduce inflammation in your throat. The addition of honey provides a gentle coating and extra anti-inflammatory properties. If you're interested, you can also use this recipe to make a calming tea.

Ingredients

I cup boiling water

I teaspoon minced fresh or dried ginger

I teaspoon honey

Steps

Transfer the hot water into a spacious mug. Include the ginger and honey, cover the mug, and let the mixture steep for I0 minutes.

Allow the liquid to cool to room temperature or refrigerate it for a cooler experience. Take I tablespoon at a time and repeat as necessary to soothe throat irritation. Keep refrigerated for up to 3 days.

Menopause

Menopause is a natural transition in female hormone function, but regrettably, it often comes with physical discomfort. Aside from these natural remedies, incorporating regular physical activity and consuming a diet rich in non-GMO soy, a natural source of plant estrogen, can also be beneficial.

Fennel-Sage Decoction

Makes I cup

This fennel and sage decoction provides estrogenic properties and can be helpful in managing hot flashes when they occur. You have the option to make a larger batch if you prefer, and you can store it in the refrigerator for up to a week for convenience. You may consider adding a sweetener to enhance the flavor, if desired.

Ingredients

2 cups water

I teaspoon fennel seeds

I teaspoon sage

Steps

Combine all the ingredients in a saucepan and bring to a boil over high heat.

Lower the heat and let the mixture simmer until the liquid is reduced by half.

Allow the decoction to cool for a few minutes. Enjoy a leisurely drink of the full quantity.

Black Cohosh Tincture

Makes about 2 cups

Black cohosh contains isoflavones that imitate the hormonal activity typically found in females. It can be helpful in managing the symptoms commonly experienced during menopause, such as mild depression, vaginal dryness, and hot flashes. This tincture has a long shelf life of up to 6 years when stored in a cool, dark place.

Ingredients

8 ounces black cohosh, finely chopped

2 cups unflavored 80-proof vodka

Steps

Place the black cohosh in a sterilized pint jar. Fill the jar to the brim with vodka, ensuring that the herbs are fully submerged.

Make sure to seal the jar securely and give it a good shake. Keep it in a cool, dark cabinet and give it a gentle shake a few times each week for 6 to 8 weeks. If any of the alcohol evaporates, make sure to replenish it with more vodka until the jar is completely filled again.

Moisten a piece of cheesecloth and place it gently over the opening of a funnel. Transfer the tincture through the funnel into a clean pint jar. Extract the liquid from the herbs by firmly squeezing the cheesecloth until all the liquid has been released. Dispose of the used herbs and carefully pour the completed tincture into glass bottles with a dark hue.

Take half a teaspoon by mouth once daily. If the flavor is too intense for your liking, you have the option to dilute the tincture by mixing it into a glass of water or juice before consumption.

Mental Wellness

Challenging professions, packed agendas, and draining experiences can leave you feeling anxious, downcast, and low on energy. Using herbs can have a significant impact, but it's important to prioritize safety and always consult your doctor before making any changes to your prescription medication.

St. John's Wort Tea

Makes I cup

While this remedy is simple and straightforward, it is highly effective for managing anxiety and minor depression. If tea isn't your cup of tea, consider trying a top-notch St. John's wort supplement and follow the recommended dosage.

Ingredients

I cup boiling water

I teaspoon dried St. John's wort

Steps

Pour the boiling water into a large mug. Add the St. John's wort, cover the mug, and allow the tea too steep for 10 minutes.

Relax and drink the tea slowly while inhaling the steam. Repeat up to two times per day.

Chamomile-Passionflower Decoction

Makes I cup

Chamomile and passionflower are known for their calming properties, helping to promote relaxation and alleviate anxiety. This blend is incredibly calming and can assist in achieving a more restful sleep, particularly during times of worry-induced insomnia. Feel free to enhance the flavor if you prefer.

Ingredients

2 cups water

1 teaspoon dried chamomile

1 teaspoon dried passionflower

Steps

Combine all the ingredients in a saucepan and bring to a boil over high heat.

Lower the heat and let the mixture simmer until the liquid is reduced by half.

Allow the decoction to cool for 5 to 10 minutes. Enjoy a leisurely drink of the full quantity.

Precautions: Avoid chamomile if you have allergies to plants in the ragweed family or if you are on prescription blood thinners. Avoid using passionflower if you are pregnant or if you have baldness or prostate problems.

Muscle Cramps

The discomfort and muscle contractions that accompany tight muscles can hinder your normal movement and even disrupt your sleep.
Using herbs can provide relief from muscle tension and promote rest for the body's healing process. If you frequently experience cramps, it is advisable to consult your doctor, as they could be indicative of an underlying medical condition.

Rosemary Liniment

Makes ½ cup

Rosemary has the ability to enhance circulation and contains components that can alleviate discomfort. Enhance the potency of this straightforward solution by incorporating rosemary essential oil. When stored in the refrigerator, the product will remain fresh for a remarkable 7 years.

Ingredients

2 tablespoons rosemary tincture

⅓ Cup unflavored 80-proof vodka

20 drops rosemary essential oil (optional)

Steps

In a dark-colored glass bottle, combine the ingredients by shaking gently.

With a cotton cosmetic pad, apply 5 to 10 drops to the cramped area. Use a little more or less as needed.

Repeat hourly while having cramps or muscle spasms.

Ginger Salve

Makes about I cup

Ginger enhances blood circulation and provides a warming sensation that deeply penetrates the skin.

Its exceptional anti-inflammatory and pain-relieving properties make it an excellent choice for addressing muscle cramps.

Ingredients

2 ounces dry or freeze-dried gingerroot, chopped

I cup light olive oil

I ounce beeswax

Steps

Combine the ginger and olive oil in a slow cooker. Choose the lowest heat setting, cover the slow cooker, and let the ginger steep in the oil for 3 to 5 hours. Switch off the heat and let the infused oil cool down.

Bring a small amount of water to a gentle simmer in the base of a double boiler.

Lower the heat to a lower setting.

Place a cheesecloth over the top of the double boiler. Add the infused oil, then squeeze and twist the cheesecloth until all the oil is extracted.

Dispose of the cheesecloth and used herbs.

Combine the beeswax with the infused oil and carefully position the double boiler on the base.

Warm slowly over low heat. Once the beeswax has melted completely, carefully take the pan off the heat. Efficiently transfer the salve into pristine, dry jars or tins and let it cool entirely before sealing.

Gently massage a small amount into the cramped area using your fingertips.

Adjust the amount as necessary and repeat as needed if cramping occurs.

Precautions: Do not use ginger if you take prescription blood thinners, have gallbladder disease, or have a bleeding disorder.

Oily Skin

Excessive sebum production leads to oily skin, as it is responsible for moisturizing and waterproofing the skin. Aggressive treatments may excessively dry out your skin and actually stimulate more sebum production, exacerbating the issue rather than improving it. Take a gentle approach to caring for your oily skin, and achieving balance will become much easier.

Rosemary Toner

Makes about 1 cup

Rosemary is a gentle astringent that helps balance skin. The witch hazel that serves as the base for this toner refreshes your skin without drying it out. This toner stays fresh for up to 6 months when stored in the refrigerator.

Ingredients

1 cup witch hazel

2 tablespoons rosemary tincture

Steps

Combine the ingredients by gently shaking them in a dark-colored glass bottle.

Using a cotton cosmetic pad, gently apply a small amount to your face. Adjust the amount as necessary.

Repeat twice daily or whenever you want to rejuvenate your skin.

Peppermint Scrub

Makes I cup

Peppermint provides a soothing and refreshing sensation to the skin, leaving it clean and revitalized. This recipe contains gentle ingredients and can be used on a daily basis, if desired. This scrub can remain fresh for up to 2 months when stored in a cool, dry place.

Ingredients

I cup dried peppermint leaves, packed

¾ cup baking soda

Steps

Combine the peppermint leaves and baking soda in a food processor or blender. Continue processing until a fine powder is achieved.

Move the mixture to a fresh container that has a secure lid.

Moisten your face and apply a small amount of the scrub to gently massage your skin, using gentle pressure and circular motions. Remember to rinse thoroughly after you have covered all areas. Make sure to repeat once or twice per day.

Premenstrual Syndrome (PMS)

Irritability, mood swings, bloating, and headaches are some of the most frequently experienced symptoms associated with PMS. Although it is a common experience for women to face mental and physical discomfort before their monthly period, it can be quite challenging. These remedies are effective in alleviating the symptoms.

Dandelion-Ginger Tea

Makes I cup

Dandelion helps alleviate bloating that can occur during PMS, while ginger provides relief for cramps and uplifts your mood. If you enjoy the flavor of this tea and wish to indulge in it more often, preparing a generous amount is a simple task. Store it in a pitcher in the refrigerator, and it will remain fresh for up to a week.

Ingredients

I cup boiling water

I teaspoon chopped dandelion root

I teaspoon chopped gingerroot

Steps

Transfer the hot water into a spacious mug. Include the roots, place a lid on the mug, and let the tea steep for 10 minutes.

Take your time and savor the tea as you enjoy the soothing steam. Can be repeated up to four times per day.

Precautions: Avoid using ginger if you are currently taking prescription blood thinners, have gallbladder disease, or suffer from a bleeding disorder.

Black Cohosh Syrup

Makes about 2 cups

Black cohosh can assist in regulating hormonal activity, providing some relief from PMS symptoms. This syrup has a slightly bitter taste and is a convenient substitute for tea. It can be stored in the refrigerator for up to 6 months.

Ingredients

2 ounces black cohosh

2 cups water

1 cup honey

Steps

Combine the black cohosh and water in a saucepan. Simmer the liquid over low heat, covering it partially with a lid, until it is reduced by half.

Pour the contents of the saucepan into a glass measuring cup, and then strain the mixture back into the saucepan using a dampened piece of cheesecloth. Squeeze the cheesecloth until no more liquid is extracted.

Include the honey and gently heat the mixture on a low flame, stirring continuously and ceasing when the temperature reaches 105°F to 110°F.

Transfer the syrup into a sterilized jar or bottle and keep it in the refrigerator.

Administer 1 tablespoon orally three times per day when experiencing PMS symptoms.

Ringworm

Contrary to its name, ringworm is not caused by a parasite. On the contrary, it is a fungal infection that manifests as red, circular patches with raised, blister-like edges. Ringworm is a highly contagious and extremely itchy condition that can easily spread from person to person, and even affect your pets. It is important to maintain proper hygiene if you contract it, and ensure that the affected area remains clean and dry while antifungal herbs are being used.

Fresh Garlic Compress

Makes I compress

Garlic is an effective antifungal agent that efficiently combats ringworm. If you happen to experience an itching and tingling sensation in a specific area without any visible rash, one possible solution is to apply fresh garlic to that spot. This may help prevent the rash from developing.

Ingredients

I cup steaming-hot water (not boiling)

I garlic clove, cut in half

Steps

Immerse a gentle cloth in the warm water.

Mash or blend half of the garlic clove and spread the paste onto the area. Place the cloth over it and secure it with a bandage to keep the treatment in place.

If you're in a hurry, place half of the garlic clove over the ringworm rash with the cut side facing down. Place the cloth over it and secure it with a bandage.

Keep the compress on for 10 to 15 minutes, then remove the garlic.

It is recommended to use a fresh piece of garlic for each affected area of ringworm.

Continue the treatment two or three times per day until the ringworm is completely eliminated.

Precautions: Garlic can cause skin irritation in sensitive individuals.

Discontinue use if this occurs.

Goldenseal Balm

Makes ½ cup

Goldenseal is a powerful antifungal agent that can provide relief from the itching caused by ringworm. It also has anti-inflammatory properties that can help reduce inflammation. This recipe contains coconut oil, which has antifungal properties and can promote faster healing of the skin. If you happen to have tea tree essential oil available, incorporating it into this recipe will enhance the potency of the balm.

Ingredients

2 ounces dried goldenseal root

¼ cup coconut oil

½ ounce beeswax

20 drops tea tree essential oil (optional)

Steps

Combine the goldenseal and coconut oil in a slow cooker. Choose the lowest heat setting, cover the slow cooker, and let the herbs steep in the oil for 3 to 5 hours. Disable the heat and let the infused oil cool down.

Bring a small amount of water to a gentle simmer in the base of a double boiler.

Lower the heat to a lower setting.

Place a piece of cheesecloth over the top portion of the double boiler. Add the infused oil and squeeze the cheesecloth until all the oil has been extracted.

Dispose of the used herbs.

Combine the beeswax with the infused oil and carefully position the double boiler on the base.

Warm slowly over low heat. Once the beeswax has melted completely, carefully take the pan off the heat. If you choose to use it, add the tea tree essential oil. Efficiently transfer the salve into pristine, dry jars or tins and let it cool entirely before sealing.

Using a cotton cosmetic pad or gauze pad, gently apply a small amount of the balm to the affected areas where ringworm is a concern. Apply three or four times a day, with a final application before going to bed. Continue the treatment until the ringworm has completely cleared.

Sore Muscles

Typically resulting from excessive exertion or prolonged periods of immobility, sore muscles require time to recover. Using herbs can provide relief and promote relaxation, while allowing yourself to rest for a day or two can speed up the healing process.

Ginger-Fennel Massage Oil

Makes I cup

Fennel and ginger provide a delightful, comforting sensation that eases and calms tense, achy muscles. This treatment will remain fresh for up to 6 months when stored in a cool, dark place.

Ingredients

I tablespoon crushed fennel seeds

2 ounces dried gingerroot, chopped

I cup light olive oil

Steps

Combine the fennel, ginger, and olive oil in a slow cooker. Choose the lowest heat setting, cover the slow cooker, and let the herbs steep in the oil for 3 to 5 hours. Switch off the heat and let the infused oil cool down.

Place a piece of cheesecloth gently over a bowl. Add the infused oil and squeeze the cheesecloth tightly until all the oil has been extracted. Remove the cheesecloth and used herbs.

Move the oil into a container that is dark in color and has a lid that fits securely.

Using your fingertips, gently apply a teaspoon of the oil to the areas that need it, adjusting the amount as necessary. Massage with a touch of intensity. Use as frequently as necessary to offer pain relief without the use of medication.

Peppermint–St. John's Wort Salve

Makes about I cup

Peppermint and St. John's wort offer effective pain relief and promote muscle relaxation. Take caution when using this remedy once it's complete, as the vibrant hue of the St. John's wort may leave stains on clothing. When properly stored, this salve can maintain its freshness for up to a year.

Ingredients

I cup light olive oil

2 ounces St. John's wort

I ounce dried peppermint

I ounce beeswax

Steps

Combine the olive oil, St. John's wort, and peppermint in a slow cooker.

Choose the lowest heat setting, cover the slow cooker, and let the herbs steep in the oil for 3 to 5 hours. Switch off the heat and let the infused oil cool down.

Heat a small amount of water in the base of a double boiler until it simmers.

Lower the heat to a gentle simmer.

Place a piece of cheesecloth over the top section of the double boiler. Add the infused oil, then squeeze and twist the cheesecloth until all the oil has been extracted. Dispose of the cheesecloth and used herbs.

Combine the beeswax with the infused oil and carefully position the double boiler on the base.

Warm slowly over low heat. Once the beeswax has completely melted, carefully take the mixture off the heat. Efficiently transfer the salve into pristine, dry jars or tins and let it cool entirely before sealing.

Using your fingertips, apply a small amount of the salve to the affected area, adjusting the quantity as necessary. Feel free to repeat as often as necessary to experience relief from pain.

Sore Throat

Regardless of the cause of your sore throat, the discomfort can be quite unpleasant and leave you feeling miserable. While herbal remedies can be effective, antibiotics may be necessary if a bacterial infection is present. If you suspect that strep throat is the cause, it is important to promptly schedule an appointment with your doctor.

Peppermint Tea with Comfrey and Sage

Makes I cup

Peppermint, comfrey, and sage are known for their soothing properties that can help alleviate the discomfort of a sore throat. The comforting warmth of the tea also offers extra relief by reducing inflammation. If you feel that the taste of this tea is too strong for your liking, you can add honey and lemon to adjust the flavor to your preference.

Ingredients

I cup boiling water

I teaspoon dried peppermint

I teaspoon dried comfrey

I teaspoon dried sage

Steps

Transfer the hot water into a spacious mug. Include the dried herbs, place a lid on the mug, and let the tea steep for 10 minutes.

Take a deep breath and enjoy the soothing tea. Use as directed, up to four times per day as necessary.

Agrimony-Licorice Gargle

Makes I cup

Agrimony, licorice, and honey offer a comforting solution for pain relief. If you prefer, you have the option to enjoy this gargle as a tea. If you prefer a refreshing experience, you can refrigerate it before using.

Ingredients

I cup boiling water

I tablespoon agrimony

I teaspoon chopped licorice root

I teaspoon honey

Steps

Transfer the hot water into a spacious mug. Include the herbs and honey, place a lid on the mug, and let the mixture steep for 10 minutes.

Allow the liquid to cool to room temperature. Take I tablespoon at a time and repeat as necessary to alleviate throat discomfort.

Sunburn

Although it's ideal to prevent sunburn, even cautious individuals can still experience it. If you're struggling to sleep due to discomfort, you may want to try incorporating a herbal sedative alongside the topical remedies mentioned in this guide. If your sunburn is severe, with blisters, serious pain, or signs of infection, it is important to seek medical attention.

Comfrey Spray

Makes about 1 cup

This fast-acting comfrey spray provides rapid relief for sunburns, thanks to the soothing properties of the comfrey tincture and witch hazel. When stored in a cool environment, it will remain fresh for up to a year.

Ingredients

1 cup witch hazel

2 tablespoons comfrey tincture

Steps

Mix the witch hazel and comfrey tincture in a glass bottle with a spray top. Gently shake to blend thoroughly.

Apply 1 or 2 spritzes to each sunburned area, adjusting the amount as necessary.

Make sure to let the spray dry completely before getting dressed, and opt for comfortable, lightweight clothing.

Repeat three or four times daily until your sunburn heals.

Hyssop-Infused Aloe Vera Gel

Makes about ½ cup

Hyssop and aloe vera gel are effective in soothing sunburns and aiding in the healing process. If you prefer not to go through the process of making a hyssop decoction and happen to have hyssop tincture available, you can substitute I tablespoon of it for the infusion. This gel can remain fresh for up to 2 weeks when stored in the refrigerator.

Ingredients

2 tablespoons dried hyssop

½ cup water

¼ cup aloe vera gel

Steps

Combine the hyssop and water in a saucepan. Bring the mixture to a rapid boil over high heat, then lower the heat to a gentle simmer. Cook the mixture until it reduces by half, then take it off the heat and let it cool completely.

Moisten a piece of cheesecloth and place it gently over the opening of a funnel. Transfer the mixture through the funnel into a glass bowl. Extract the liquid from the herbs by firmly squeezing the cheesecloth until all the liquid has been released.

Combine the aloe vera gel with the liquid and mix it together using a whisk. Place the completed gel into a sterilized glass jar. Make sure to seal the jar securely and place it in the refrigerator.

Using a cotton cosmetic pad or your fingertips, gently apply a thin layer to the affected areas three or four times per day.

Weight Loss

Obesity is a chronic condition that goes beyond mere appearance. It can exacerbate other illnesses while causing discomfort in your own skin. It's absolutely true that maintaining a healthy, whole-foods diet and incorporating regular exercise are crucial for achieving and sustaining weight loss. It's worth noting that incorporating herbs into your routine can help facilitate a smoother transition to a healthier lifestyle and support a more efficient metabolism.

Dieter's Tea Blend with Chickweed, Dandelion, and Fennel

Makes I cup

Chickweed, dandelion, and fennel can aid in weight loss by eliminating toxins and reducing bloating and water retention. Fennel can assist in reducing your appetite, making it somewhat more manageable to resist cravings. This tea blend will remain fresh for up to 2 months when stored in a cool, dry place. If you prefer, you have the option to enhance the flavor of your hot tea with a touch of lemon juice.

Ingredients

3 ounces dried chickweed

3 ounces dried dandelion root, chopped

3 ounces fennel seeds, crushed

I cup boiling water

Steps

Combine the chickweed, dandelion root, and fennel in a large container with a tight-fitting lid.

Measure two teaspoons of the tea mixture into a large mug. Simply add the boiling water, cover the mug, and let the herbs steep for 10 minutes.

Enjoy a cup of tea. Indulge in two or three cups per day to support your weight loss journey.

Ginseng Tincture

Makes about 2 cups

Ginseng offers numerous benefits such as improved circulation, enhanced mood, and nutritional support during weight loss. This is an excellent source of vitamin B12, which is essential for the production of red blood cells and converting food into energy. This tincture is an excellent overall tonic that will maintain its freshness for up to 6 years when stored in a cool, dry place.

Ingredients

8 ounces Panax ginseng or American ginseng, finely chopped

2 cups unflavored 80-proof vodka

Steps

Put the ginseng in a sterilized pint jar. Add the vodka, filling the jar to the very top and covering the herbs completely.

Cap the jar tightly and shake it up. Store it in a cool, dark cabinet and shake it several times per week for 6 to 8 weeks. If any of the alcohol evaporates, add more vodka so that the jar is again full to the top.

Dampen a piece of cheesecloth and drape it over the mouth of a funnel. Pour the tincture through the funnel into another sterilized pint jar. Squeeze the liquid from the herbs, wringing the cheesecloth until no more liquid comes out. Discard the spent herbs and transfer the finished tincture to dark-colored glass bottles.

Take ½ teaspoon orally each morning for 1 month, and then take 2 weeks off from the remedy. Repeat this cycle as many times as you like.

Chapter 4

Important Herbs to Familiarize Yourself With

Here you'll find a wide range of herbal medicine staples, including agrimony and witch hazel. This list does not include all the common herbs available, as there are numerous safe and beneficial ones to explore. However, these options are incredibly easy to use. All of them are available for purchase in their complete form, and many can be easily found in various convenient forms such as capsules, salves, tablets, teas, tinctures, and more.

Agrimony

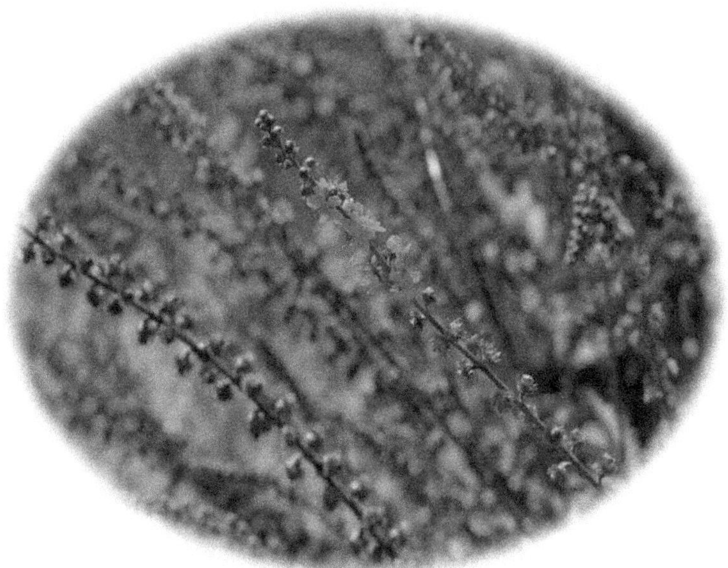

Agrimonia eupatoria, Agrimonia gryposepala

In the past, agrimony was frequently used to address coughs, diarrhea, skin issues, and sore throats. This herb is quite popular and has a pleasant aroma that may bring to mind the scent of apricots. It is a delightful complement to herbal teas, particularly when you are feeling under the weather with a cold or the flu.

Parts Used: Leaves and flowers

Precautions: Can aggravate constipation

Identifying/Growing: Agrimony, also known as the cocklebur or sticklewort, belongs to the rose family. Its woody stem is covered in soft down, rather than prickly thorns. The branches are adorned with toothy, dark green leaves, which eventually give way to spikes of small, bright yellow flowers that leave prickly burrs behind as they fade. The plant typically grows to an average height of 2 feet, although some plants can reach up to 4 feet.

Although agrimony is commonly found in fields and woodlands throughout Europe and North America, it is quite easy to grow. It thrives in sunny conditions and benefits from regular watering. It is important to maintain the soil's moisture and ensure proper drainage.

Feel free to harvest the leaves at any point during the season, and simply snip the flowers once they start to bloom.

Aloe

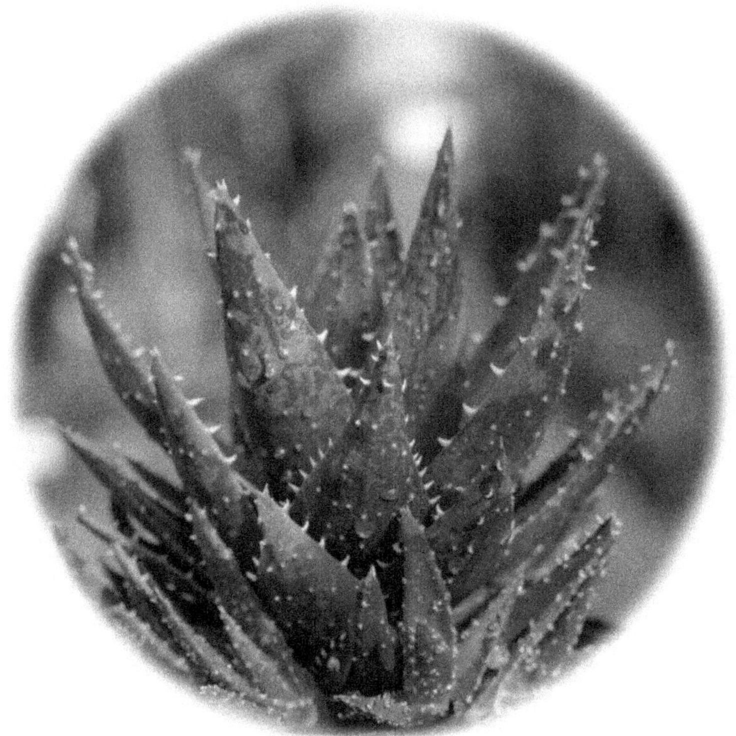

Aloe vera, Aloe barbadensis, Aloe ferox

Despite its resemblance to a cactus, aloe actually belongs to the lily family. The thick, spiky leaves contain a gel that has healing properties and can be used to treat burns, cuts, and scrapes. While fresh aloe is great to have available, the bottled version is also highly effective and convenient.

Parts Used: Gel and juice from inner leaves

Precautions: Aloe juice is a strong laxative. It should not be taken internally during pregnancy or while breastfeeding.

Identifying/Growing: There are more than 250 aloe species found across the globe. The majority of species originate from Africa and showcase beautiful gray-green leaf patterns. They also have tall, slender stems that produce yellow, tube-shaped flowers. This plant is not commonly found in the wild, unless you reside in a tropical climate. However, it can be effortlessly cultivated as an indoor plant.

Choose a spacious container and use well-draining soil when planting your aloe. Provide it with slow-release pellets or a 10-40-10 fertilizer, and make sure to water it consistently. Make sure to let the soil dry completely between waterings, especially in the winter months when it goes into its dormant phase. If you reside in a chilly region that experiences hot summers, you are welcome to place your aloe vera plants outside when there is no risk of freezing temperatures.

Angelica

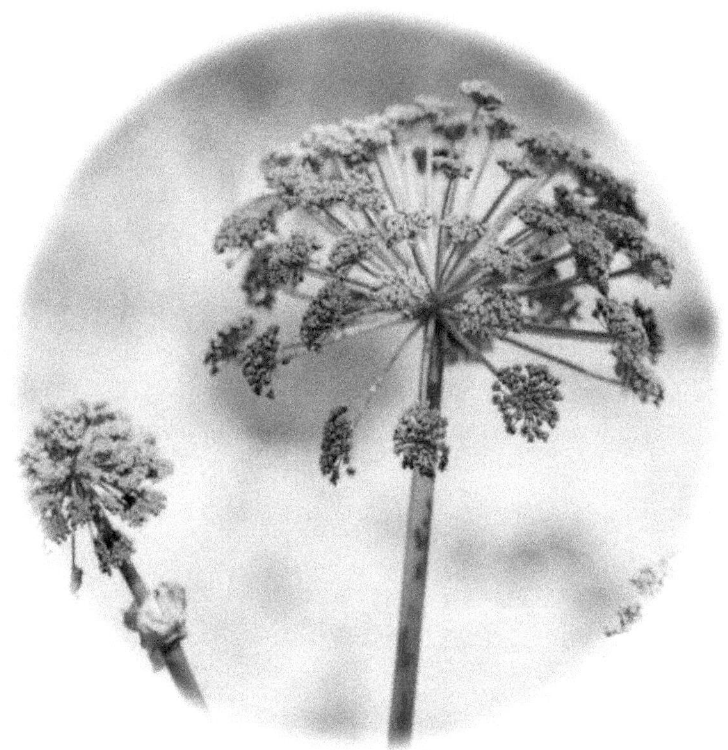

Angelica archangelica

Angelica has a long history of being used as a natural remedy to help induce labor in cases of delayed childbirth. This herb is highly effective in providing relief for painful menstruation and cramps. Additionally, its capacity to alleviate congestion and indigestion makes it a valuable option for addressing the needs of the entire family.

Parts Used: Root, leaves, stems, and fruit

Precautions: Angelica has the ability to enhance blood circulation in the pelvic area and uterus, potentially leading to the initiation of menstruation. It is not recommended for use during pregnancy. This product has elevated levels of coumarin, an organic compound known for its pleasant fragrance and ability to thin the blood. It is important to note that this may potentially interact negatively with anticoagulant medications.

Identifying/Growing: Angelica can be found growing freely in fields and meadows across temperate zones worldwide, especially near streams and rivers. It thrives in partially shaded areas, reaching a height of 3 to 6 feet. A delightful fragrance fills the air as clusters of small, creamy yellow or greenish flowers bloom in late June to July.

Angelica can thrive in a variety of lighting conditions, ranging from partial shade to full sun. Moist, well-drained soil is recommended, along with being close to a water feature. Ensure proper spacing between your plants after germination, allowing them enough room to grow. Only harvest your plants once they have reached full maturity.

Angelica is a biennial plant. By planting it consecutively each year, you can guarantee a yearly harvest.

Arnica

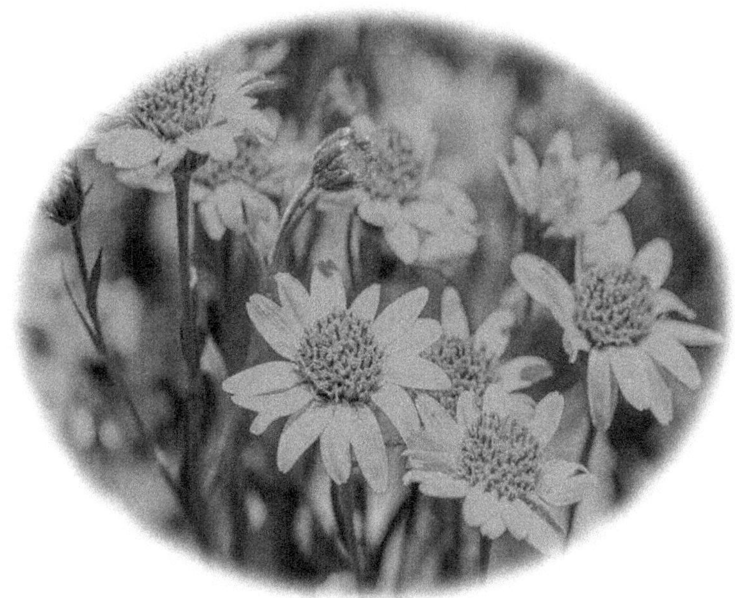

Arnica Montana

Arnica is a stunning alpine herb that possesses remarkable anti-inflammatory properties, making it widely recognized beyond the realm of herbal medicine. Although arnica creams and oils are convenient, you can easily find the whole herb online.

Parts Used: Flowers

Precautions: Do not use in open or bleeding wounds. Long-term use can cause skin irritation.

Identifying/Growing: This aromatic herb, also known as mountain arnica, can be found growing in alpine meadows. The plant showcases fragrant toothed leaves and vibrant yellow to orange flowers, resembling daisies, on stems that typically reach a height of 1 to 2 feet. Arnica thrives in bright sunlight, although it can also tolerate some shade. If you choose to cultivate this herb, it requires a certain level of patience as the seeds can take anywhere from 1 month to 2 years to germinate. You have two options: you can both sow the seeds outside in late summer and hope for the best, or you can sow them in large pots indoors. They will germinate at a temperature of about 55°F. Once the arnica starts growing, it will bloom and propagate through its roots and self-seeding. By trimming the plants once they have bloomed, you can often enjoy another round of blossoms. Maintain the health of your arnica by periodically dividing the plants at the roots every 3 years, either in the spring or autumn.

Basil

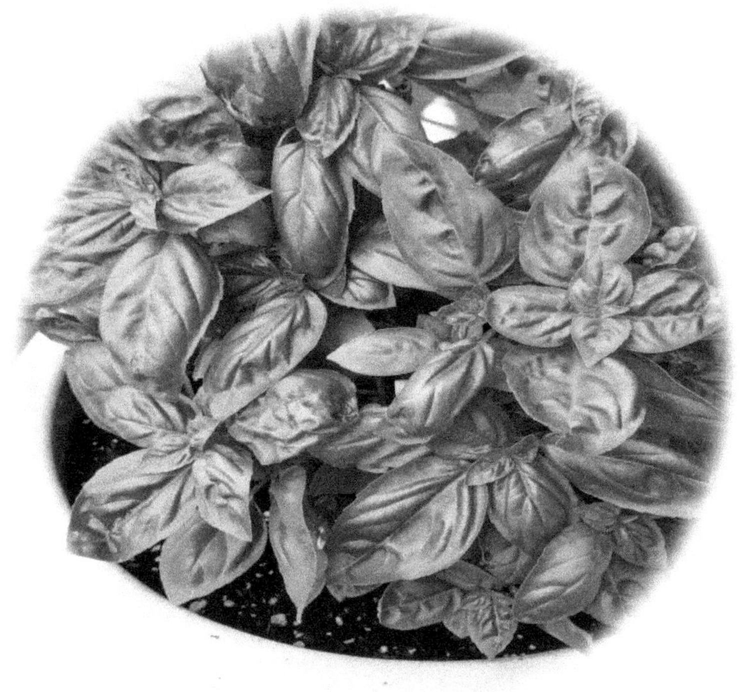

Ocimum basilicum

Many individuals are well-acquainted with the way basil can enhance the taste of food, as well as its unmistakable sweet scent. However, it's worth noting that there are numerous types of basil, each with unique antibacterial properties and the ability to soothe the stomach. Crushed fresh basil can also provide relief for insect bites.

Parts Used: Leaves

Precautions: Do not use during pregnancy.

Identifying/Growing: Basil is typically available in the produce department of your local supermarket, although it is not commonly found growing wild. Given its potency and ease of cultivation, fresh basil is a herb worth considering for even the least experienced gardeners. Basil flourishes in the garden or grows just as contentedly in a pot on a sunlit windowsill. It thrives in bright conditions and flourishes in direct sunlight. Regular watering is necessary to maintain the soil's moisture level. By selectively picking the top leaves, you can promote healthy growth and discourage the plant from producing seeds.

Black cohosh

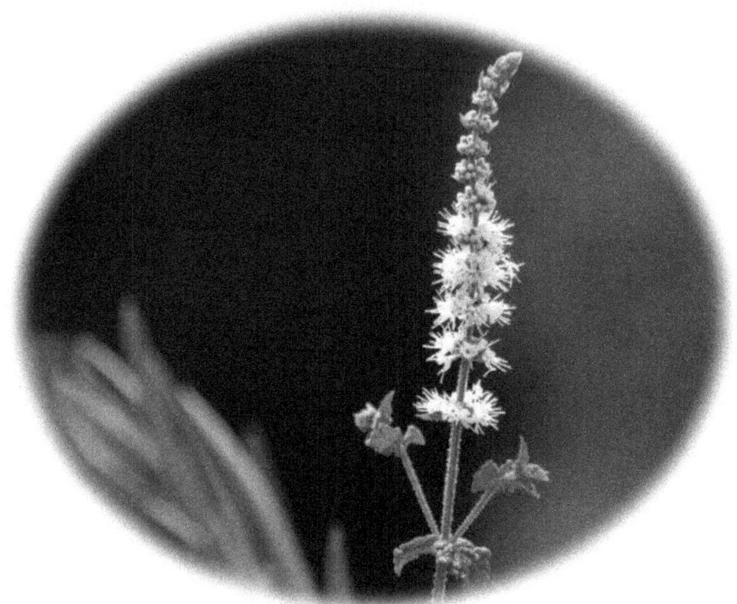

Cimicifuga racemosa

Black cohosh contains isoflavones, which have properties similar to estrogen. Black cohosh is a helpful option for managing menopause symptoms such as vaginal dryness, hot flashes, and mild depression. Additionally, it provides anti-inflammatory and pain-relieving benefits. As an effective cold and flu remedy, it effectively soothes coughs and provides relief from discomfort.

Parts Used: Root

Precautions: Do not use during pregnancy or breastfeeding. Black cohosh causes gastric discomfort in some individuals; stop using it if this occurs.

Identifying/Growing: Black cohosh is native to the eastern half of North America and tends to thrive in the outskirts of fields and open woodlands. The plant has oval-shaped leaves, tall erect stems that can reach a height of 3 feet or more, and delicate white flowers on slender spikes. Its name is derived from the dark color of its rootstock.

For optimal growth, it is recommended to plant black cohosh seeds in indoor containers during the fall season. It is important to provide them with a warm and dry environment, ideally with ample sunlight exposure. Once the plants start growing, make sure to water them on a weekly basis and keep them indoors until the risk of frost has passed. Consider relocating your black cohosh to a spot that enjoys the gentle touch of morning sunlight, while also providing a comforting shade in the afternoon. Make sure to fertilize the area with well-rotted compost before transplanting and continue this practice each spring. Make sure to water the plants regularly, especially during dry weather. If you see them starting to wilt, increase the frequency of watering.

Blue vervain

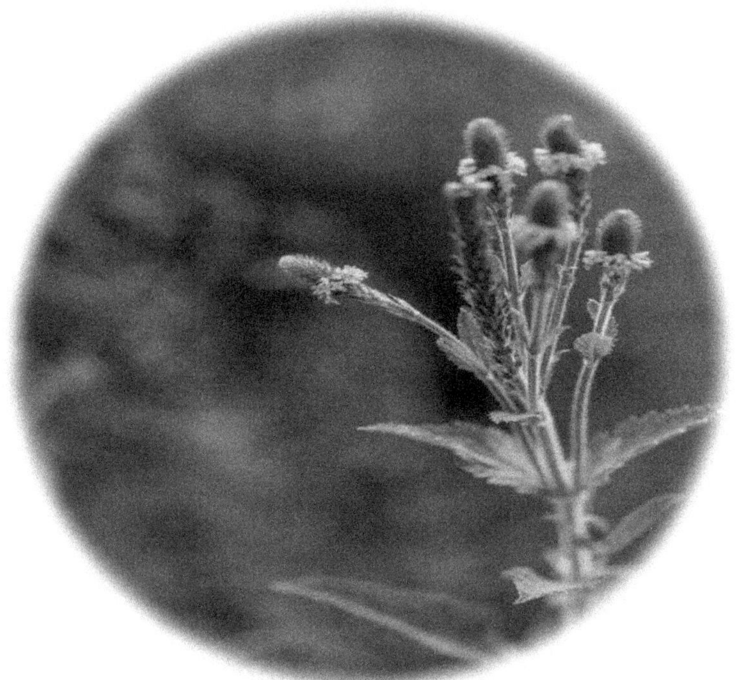

Verbena hastata, Verbena officinalis

Blue vervain is known for its ability to calm the nervous system and provide effective pain relief. It can be particularly helpful in treating conditions such as rheumatism, joint pain, and neuralgia when used in poultices. Tea leaves can provide relief for headaches, bladder discomfort, and sore throats. Next time you're dealing with chest congestion or bronchitis, consider giving blue vervain tea a try. It's known for its expectorant properties.

Parts Used: Leaves

Precautions: Do not use during pregnancy.

Identifying/Growing: Blue vervain is commonly found growing in meadows, waste places, and along roadsides across North America and Europe. The plant features lance-shaped leaves with rough, toothy edges that are arranged on stems averaging 3 to 7 feet in height. At the top of the plant, slender spikes give rise to beautiful purplish blue flowers.

This delightful herb is a breeze to cultivate. For successful germination of blue vervain, it is important to provide adequate light. To achieve this, sow the seeds and water them without covering them with soil. Remember to keep the seeds adequately watered until they begin to sprout. For more potent solutions, select the herbs prior to their blooming and promptly dry them. If you want a consistent supply year after year, you can let some of your blue vervain flower and go to seed. This way, it will self-seed and return every spring.

Catnip

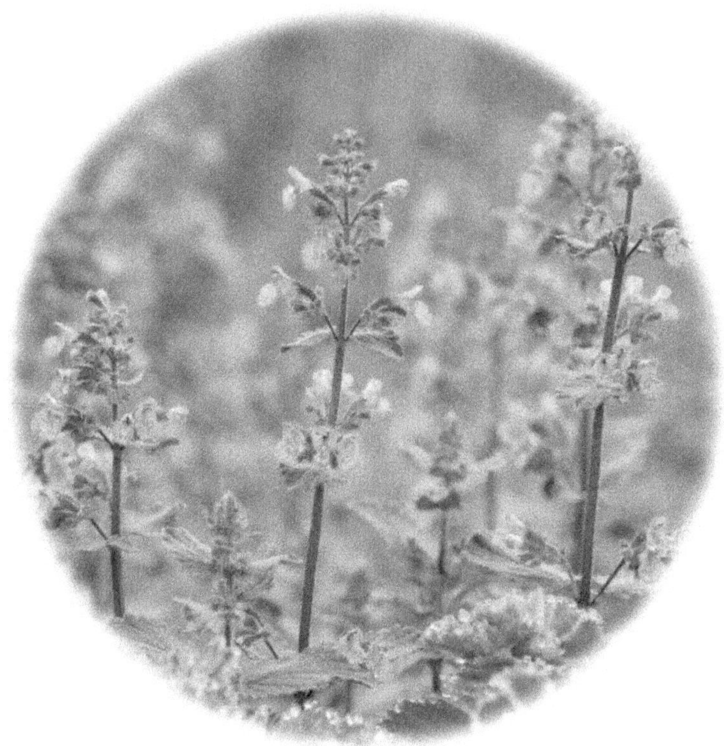

Nepeta cataria

Almost everyone is well-acquainted with catnip, a must-have indulgence for our beloved feline companions. Despite its ability to stimulate a cat's playful side, this delightful herb has the opposite effect on most individuals, encouraging Experience a state of deep relaxation without any of the negative effects commonly associated with pharmaceutical sedatives.

Parts Used: Leaves and flowering tops

Precautions: Do not use during pregnancy.

Identifying/Growing: Wild catnip can often be spotted growing alongside roads. The leaves of this plant have a delightful minty fragrance and are a lovely shade of greyish-green with a velvety texture. The upper portion of the plant is adorned with beautiful white flowers that have lavender-colored spots.

Catnip adds a lovely touch to any garden. Similar to other members of the mint family, it is effortless to cultivate and has a natural inclination to propagate if left unchecked. Begin by starting the seeds indoors during the spring season. Once the threat of frost has passed, you can then transplant the young seedlings to a sunny and well-drained location. Ensure the safety of your precious catnip plants by using a chicken wire lid to keep them out of reach from curious felines. You can enjoy the bountiful harvest of leaves and flowers season after season, year after year.

Chamomile

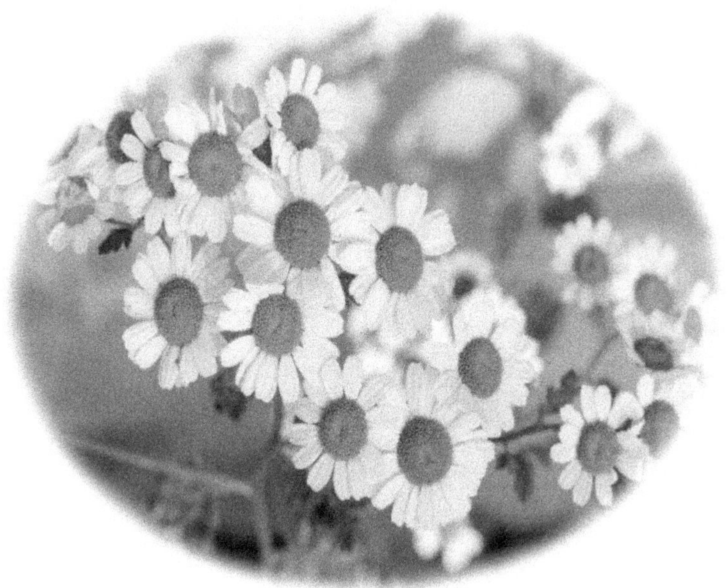

Matricaria recutita

Chamomile is known for its gentle yet effective qualities, offering antibacterial and anti-inflammatory properties. Its remarkable ability to calm the nervous system makes it an essential ingredient in tea blends designed for relaxation and sleep. Additionally, its antispasmodic properties make it a great choice for relieving tension and soothing sore muscles. Next time you're feeling stressed, sore, or having trouble sleeping, why not give chamomile a try?

Parts Used: Flowers

Precautions: Chamomile has significant levels of coumarin and may have negative interactions with blood thinners. It may also pose difficulties for individuals with ragweed allergies.

Identifying/Growing: Chamomile is originally from Europe, but it can thrive in various locations with minimal effort. The flowers of this plant are small and daisy-like, with white petals and raised yellow centers. The leaves have a delicate and feathery appearance. It's incredibly simple to cultivate from seed, creating a stunning border in the garden that effortlessly renews itself annually. Harvest the flowers when they are at their peak, and anticipate being able to enjoy two separate cuttings every summer.

Chickweed

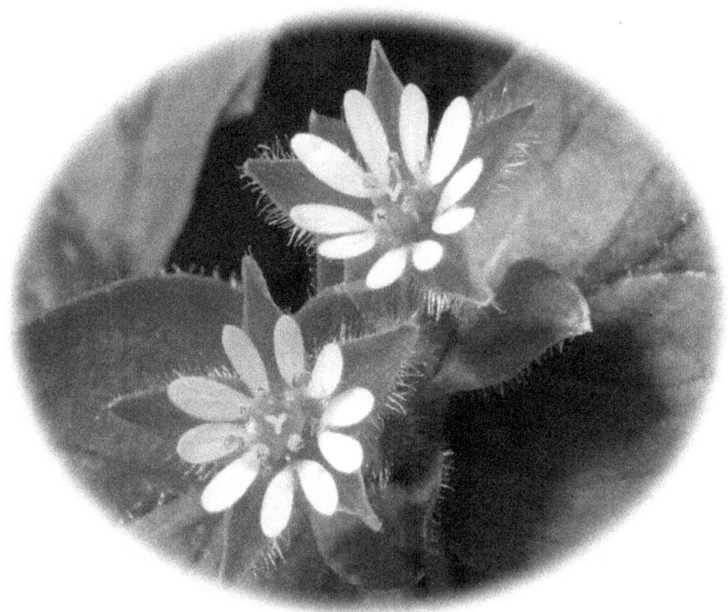

Stellaria media

Chickweed is a widely distributed wild herb that can be found in various parts of the world. You can utilize fresh chickweed to create soothing poultices for addressing rashes, irritated skin, and minor burns. Additionally, the juice can provide relief from itching. In addition to its medicinal benefits, chickweed adds a delicious touch to spring salads.

Parts Used: Leaves and flowers

Precautions: Consuming large amounts of chickweed may have a laxative effect. Take caution when foraging in locations where chemicals have been used.

Identifying/Growing: Chickweed is commonly found in lawns, as well as in wooded areas and meadows. This resilient plant thrives in various climates throughout the year, temporarily receding during freezing temperatures but promptly resurfacing at the first sign of warmth. The plant showcases delicate white flowers and oval leaves that grow from slender stems measuring around 4 to 6 inches in length.

A lot of individuals attempt to eliminate chickweed from their lawns, frequently without success.

To help it thrive, prepare a suitable area by raking the soil, ensuring it is moist, and spacing the seeds about ½ inch apart. Apply a thin layer of topsoil to the area, lightly moisten it, and allow the plants to establish themselves undisturbed. Your chickweed will naturally spread and thrive without any need for maintenance.

Comfrey

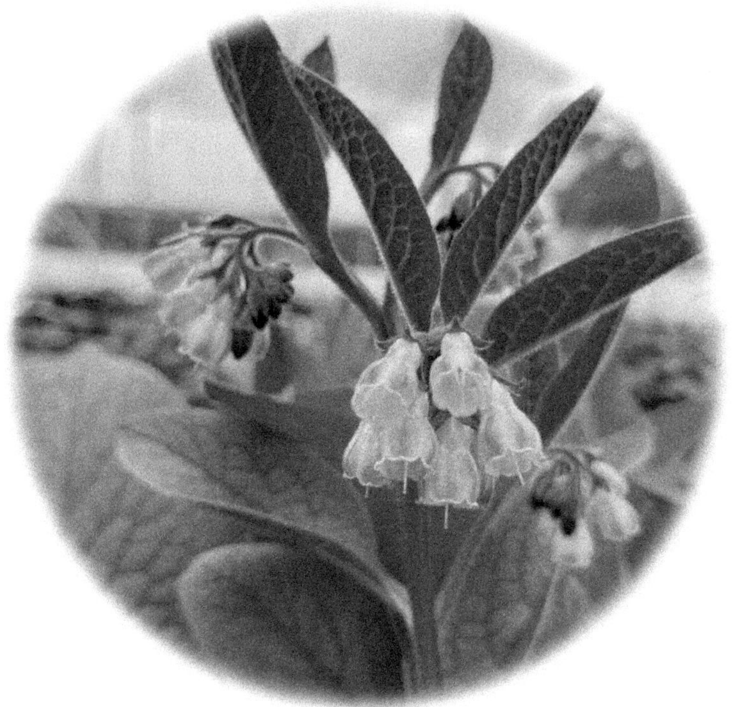

Symphytum officinale

The Latin name of comfrey is derived from the Greek word sympho, which signifies the process of promoting growth and unity. This refers to its conventional application in accelerating the healing process of fractures. The plant's remarkable effectiveness in relieving pain and inflammation is widely known. It is highly effective in treating cuts, scrapes, insect bites, burns, and rashes as well.

Parts Used: Leaves and roots

Precautions: Excessive internal use of comfrey can lead to liver damage and potentially harmful carcinogenic effects due to its natural insect-repelling pyrrolizidine alkaloids. Infants and children are particularly vulnerable, so it's important to exercise caution when deciding whether to use comfrey internally or limit it to external applications.

Identifying/Growing: Comfrey, an herbaceous perennial, is native to Europe but can thrive in partial shade in temperate to warm climates. At maturity, the plants reach impressive sizes of 3 to 6 feet in height and 2 to 4 feet in width. Comfrey's delicate hanging clusters of flowers come in various shades of pink, violet, or cream. These beautiful blooms gracefully emerge from sturdy stems adorned with large leaves. This herb is quite large, giving the impression of a shrub. However, its stems do not become woody, and the entire plant dies back during winter.

Comfrey is best cultivated through root cuttings, as they are easier to grow compared to seeds. Plant the cuttings horizontally at a depth of around 3 inches and space them approximately 3 feet apart. It flourishes in nutrient-rich soil with ample nitrogen.

Composting on a regular basis will ensure a bountiful harvest. You have the option to harvest the leaves once the plants have grown to a height of 2 feet.

Dandelion

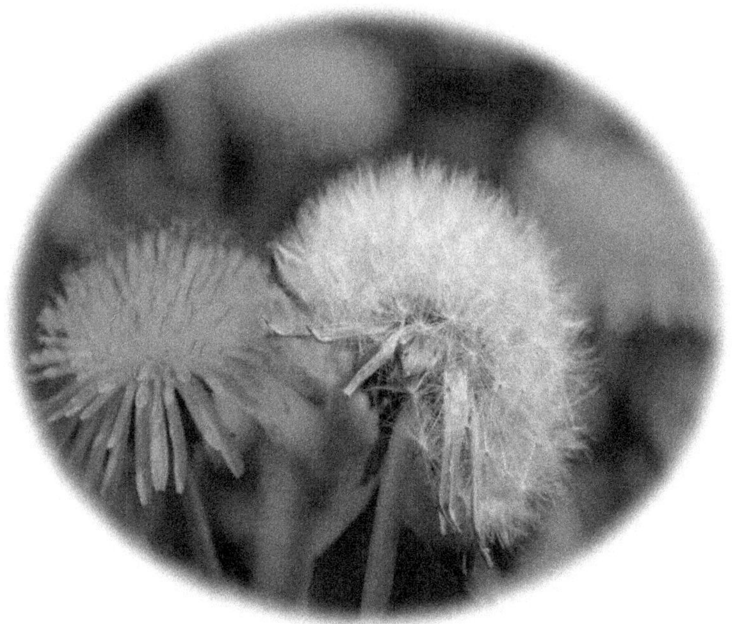

Taraxacum officinale

Dandelion is commonly seen as a pesky weed, but its liver detoxifying properties and ability to alleviate indigestion, bloating, and constipation make it a valuable plant for your garden. The root has medicinal properties, the greens are a nutritious addition to salads, and the fragrant yellow flowers attract pollinators with their nectar.

Parts Used: Roots and sap

Precautions: It is important to be cautious when harvesting dandelions to ensure they have not been exposed to any harmful chemicals like herbicides or pesticides.

Identifying/Growing: The dandelion is easily identifiable with its long, toothy leaves and fluffy, bright yellow flowers. Encouraging dandelions to populate your lawn and garden can be achieved by avoiding the use of herbicides. When harvesting roots and other plant parts, it's important to consider leaving a few plants behind and allowing them to go to seed. This way, you can ensure a bountiful supply of dandelions for the following year.

Echinacea

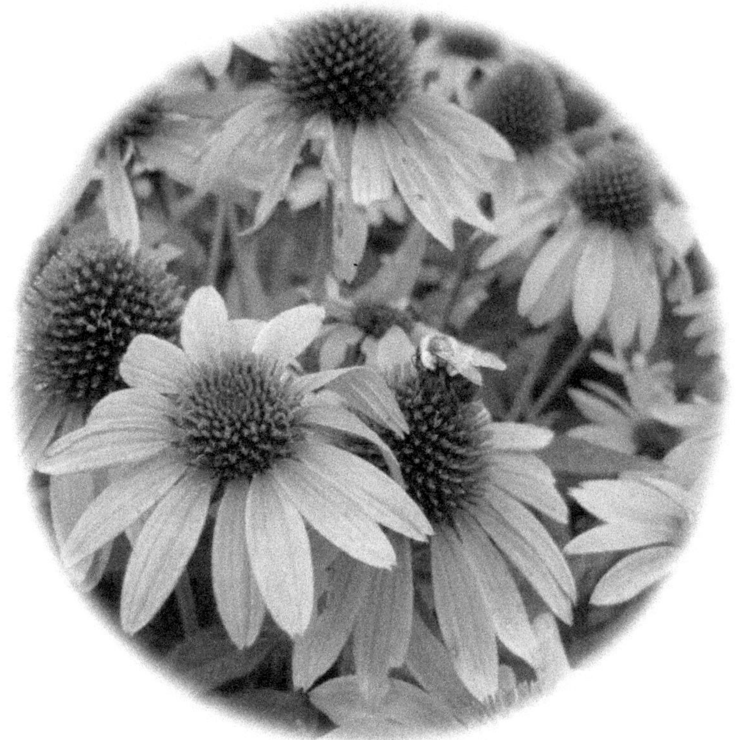

Echinacea angustifolia, Echinacea purpurea, Echinacea pallida

Echinacea has been widely used in various remedies for wound care, infection treatment, and relief from cold symptoms. When taken at the first sign of a cold or the flu, you'll notice a decrease in the duration and intensity of symptoms like coughing, fever, and sore throat. Echinacea is known for its antibacterial, antifungal, and antiviral properties, making it a valuable treatment for a range of ailments.

Parts Used: Roots

Precautions: Echinacea can potentially interact with pharmaceuticals used in immune system suppression therapy, leading to adverse reactions. It is important to avoid using echinacea if you have a chronic infection like tuberculosis or HIV/AIDS, or if you have an autoimmune disease such as lupus or rheumatoid arthritis. If Echinacea has a negative impact on you, it is advisable to discontinue its use, as it may trigger allergy symptoms in individuals with ragweed allergies.

Identifying/Growing: Echinacea, also referred to as purple coneflower, showcases striking hues of yellow, orange, and red at the heart of its daisy-like blossoms.

While echinacea is naturally found in prairies across North America, it is important to note that overharvesting has become a concern. Therefore, it is recommended to cultivate echinacea at home instead of harvesting it from the wild.

Echinacea is incredibly simple to cultivate in your garden, and in addition to providing exceptional medicinal advantages, it also has the delightful ability to attract bees and butterflies. This exquisite herb reaches a height of approximately 4 feet. If left to reproduce naturally, it will scatter its seeds and produce new shoots annually. Simply ensure that the plants have access to a sunny area with soil that is rich in lime and drains well. In return, they will bless you with their exquisite beauty and a plethora of cost-effective remedies.

Fennel

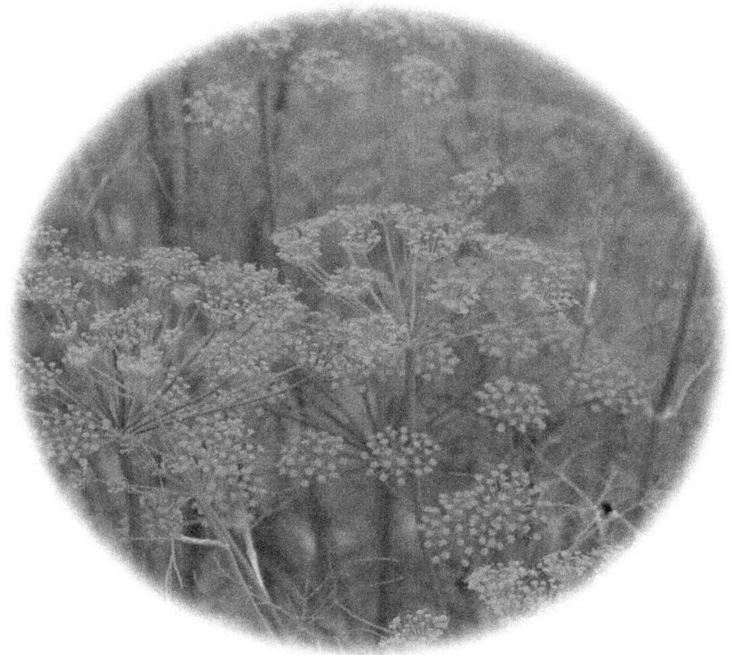

Foeniculum vulgare

Fennel, with its delightful aroma reminiscent of licorice, is a popular ingredient in kitchens around the globe. When used medicinally, the seeds of this product can provide relief from bloating, gas, and abdominal cramps. Fennel possesses properties that help regulate the female reproductive system, providing relief from menopause and menstrual symptoms.

Parts Used: Seeds

Precautions: Remedies made with seeds and other plant parts are typically safe for use. However, it is advisable to avoid using fennel essential oil if you are pregnant or breastfeeding.

Identifying/Growing: The leaves of fennel are delicate and have a beautiful dark green color. They are accompanied by vibrant green stalks that emerge from the rounded base of the plant. The base itself is ribbed and has a pale greenish-white hue. The stalks reach a maximum height of 5 feet, while the small yellow flowers grow in densely clustered formations.

Fennel thrives in sunny locations and prefers soil that drains well. Plant the seeds 12 inches apart and gently cover them with approximately ¼ inch of soil. Water the planting site gently after seeding, and ensure that the soil remains moist until shoots emerge approximately one to two weeks after planting. To prevent the plants from toppling, it is recommended to stake them once they reach a height of 18 inches.

Collect the seeds once they have turned brown, but before they naturally detach from their umbels. For a smoother process, try using cheesecloth to wrap around the top of the fennel and then cut the stalks. Make sure the seeds are thoroughly dried before placing them in a securely sealed jar.

Feverfew

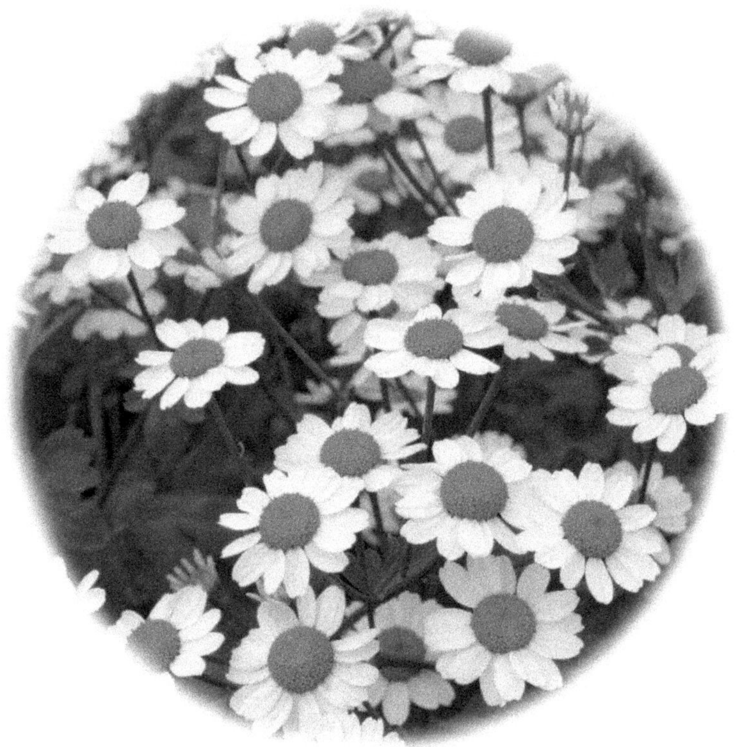

Tanacetum parthenium

Feverfew provides a gentle calming effect that is perfect for relieving the stress and exhaustion that frequently result in headaches. It helps to prevent blood platelets from sticking together in the bloodstream and keeps small capillaries from getting blocked. This action allows feverfew to effectively prevent and treat migraines.

Parts Used: Leaves

Precautions: Fresh feverfew leaves can cause mouth ulcers. Do not use feverfew during pregnancy and avoid it if you are allergic to ragweed.

Identifying/Growing: Feverfew is a close relative of marigolds and dandelions.

The flowers have small, daisy-like blooms with bright yellow centers and delicate white petals. Growing feverfew is a breeze - just plant the seeds in a sunny area during the spring or summer. When you harvest the plants, it's a good idea to leave some behind and let them go to seed. This way, you can ensure a consistent supply for the following year.

Garlic

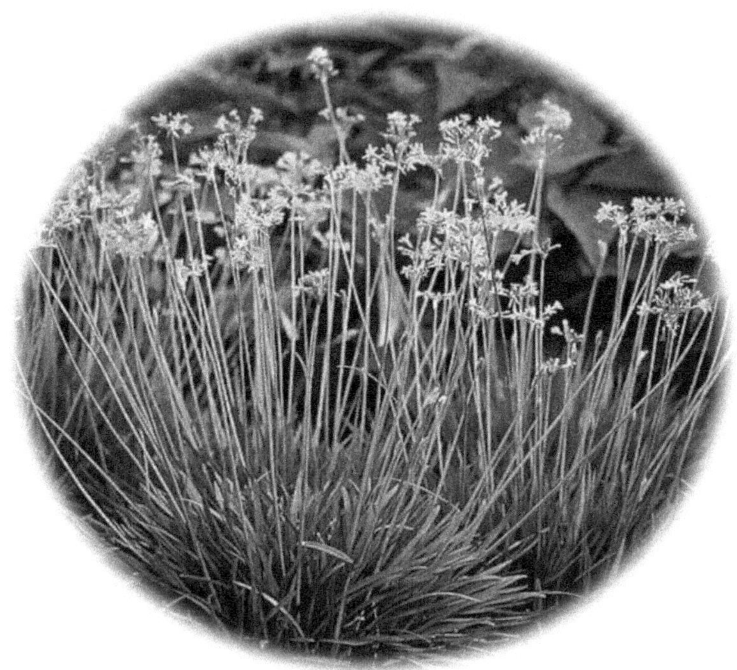

Allium sativum

Spicy garlic is a versatile ingredient that goes beyond its delicious taste, proving to be a valuable addition in various recipes. This common herb is packed with more than 30 medicinal compounds, including allicin, which is a powerful antimicrobial agent with a wide range of effectiveness. It has numerous health benefits, such as preventing blood clotting, reducing triglycerides and cholesterol levels, and supplying vital antioxidants.

Parts Used: Roots

Precautions: Overconsumption of garlic can cause gas and heartburn. When used topically, garlic can cause a skin rash in some people with sensitive skin.

Identifying/Growing: Garlic is a breeze to recognize and cultivate, and in numerous regions, you can sow it during the autumn for a bountiful springtime yield, and once more in the early spring for an additional harvest in the fall. Garlic thrives in a sunny location, where the soil has been enriched with nutrient-rich compost. Ensure that the cloves are planted with their tips facing upwards, at a depth of approximately 2 inches, and then apply a generous layer of mulch. It is important to let the soil dry out between waterings to avoid any potential rotting. Additionally, it is recommended to harvest the plant when approximately half of the leaves have turned brown or yellow.

Ginger

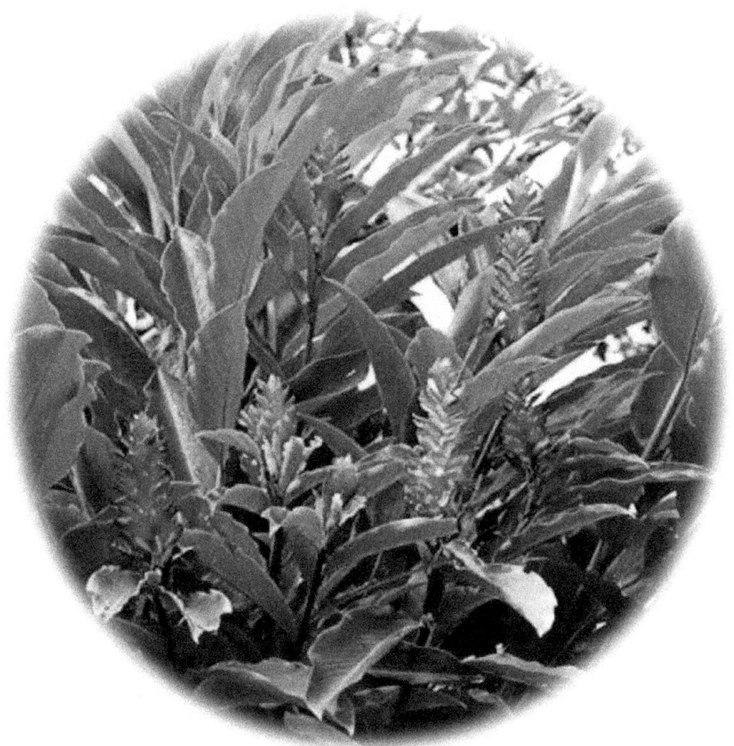

Zingiber officinale

Ginger is a versatile root that can be used in both sweet and savory dishes. It is not only delicious, but also has medicinal properties that can help with various ailments such as cramps and nausea. It has natural properties that can help thin the blood and reduce cholesterol levels. Additionally, it is known for its ability to increase body temperature and eliminate toxins, making it a valuable ingredient in cold and flu remedies.

Parts Used: Roots

Precautions: It is advisable to refrain from consuming ginger if you have a bleeding disorder or gallbladder disease, or if you are currently taking prescription blood thinners, as ginger has blood-thinning properties. When using ginger, it's important to exercise caution if you are pregnant, as it has the potential to stimulate the uterus.

Identifying/Growing: Ginger is a tropical plant that boasts waxy leaves and smooth, fragrant white flowers. When shopping at the grocery store, be sure to choose roots that have a firm texture. If you reside in a tropical climate, ginger can be cultivated outdoors. In colder areas, it can be cultivated in a greenhouse or a sunny indoor spot. For optimal growth, it is recommended to plant the roots in spacious containers, ensuring they are placed at a depth of approximately 10 inches. Ginger plants can reach impressive heights of 4 feet or more, and their blossoms emit a delightful fragrance as a reward for your hard work.

Ginkgo biloba

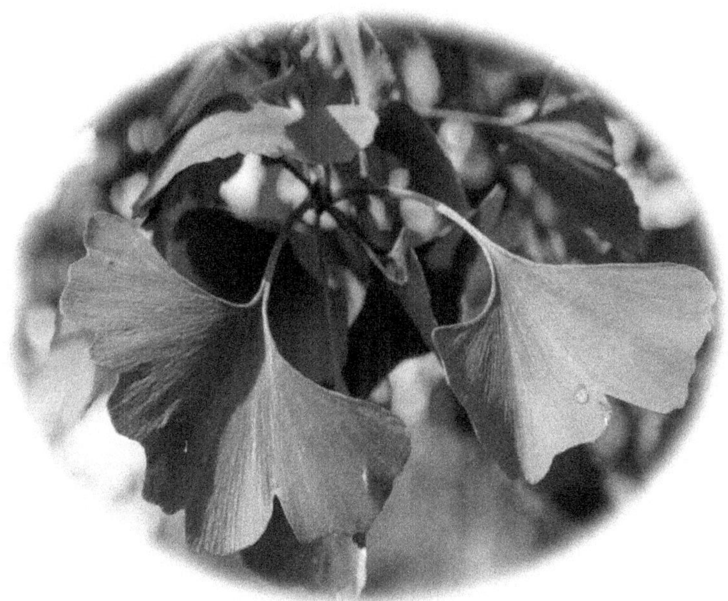

Ginkgo biloba

A stunning deciduous tree with distinctive fan-shaped leaves, ginkgo biloba promotes optimal circulation while enhancing cognitive function, sustaining your energy levels, and even boosting libido in both men and women. Ginkgo biloba is a natural option for effectively managing allergies and asthma due to its antihistamines and anti-inflammatory properties.

Parts Used: Leaves

Precautions: Avoid using ginkgo biloba if you are currently taking prescription monoamine oxidase inhibitor (MAOI) or selective serotonin reuptake inhibitor (SSRI) medications.

It is important to consult with your doctor before using Ginkgo if you are taking prescription blood thinners, as it may enhance their effects.

Identifying/Growing: Ginkgo biloba is known for its elegant trees that can reach heights of up to 100 feet. The leaves of these trees have a distinctive shape with two lobes. Ginkgo trees have an impressive lifespan of over 1,000 years, and they possess remarkable resilience against disease, insects, and pollution. In addition to their practical applications in herbal medicine, these beautiful trees can greatly enhance the aesthetic appeal of your home's landscape. Acquire a sapling from a nursery and place it in a noticeable location.

Once the tree is fully grown, you have the flexibility to harvest and utilize its vibrant leaves throughout the seasons, from spring to fall.

Goldenseal

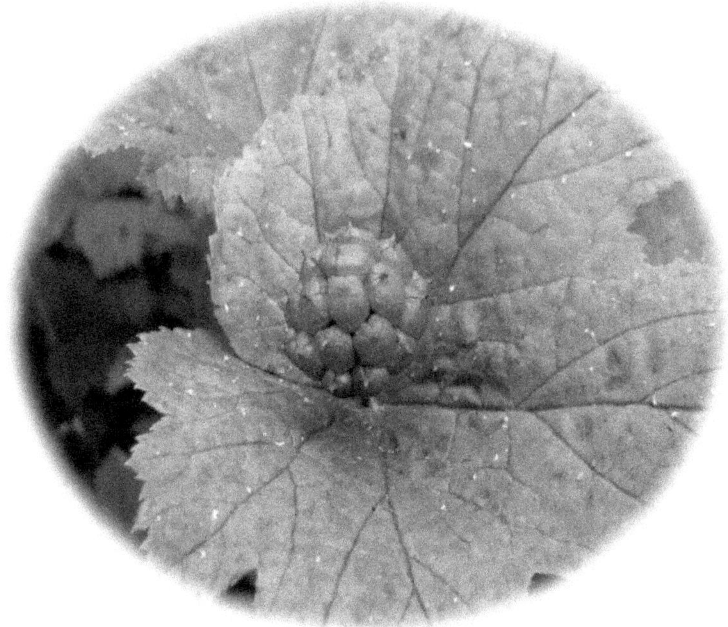

Hydrastis Canadensis

Goldenseal provides valuable antiviral and antibacterial benefits, thanks to its high levels of hydrastine and berberine. An essential herb to have readily available for various purposes, goldenseal is commonly used in remedies for cuts and wounds, sinus infections, respiratory congestion, sore throats, and other ailments.

Parts Used: Roots, primarily; leaves offer milder benefits

Precautions: Avoid the use of goldenseal if you are currently pregnant or breastfeeding, or if you have been diagnosed with high blood pressure. Goldenseal tincture may lead to stomach irritation, so it is advisable to discontinue internal use if such symptoms arise.

Identifying/Growing: Once, the lush forests from Minnesota to Georgia were home to thriving populations of wild goldenseal. Sadly, the loss of their natural habitat and excessive harvesting have caused a significant decline in their numbers.

These perennial shrubs grow to a maximum height of just 10 inches, with leaves and berries that resemble those of the raspberry. The roots have a thick and knotted appearance, and their interiors are a vibrant shade of yellow.

Growing goldenseal requires a protected area with deep, loamy soil and dappled shade. The rootstock can be divided into sections that are at least ½ inch in size. These sections should be placed about 8 inches apart and buried at a depth of 2 to 3 inches. Make sure to plant the rhizomes during the autumn season and maintain a well-mulched and weed-free area.

Goldenseal has a rather leisurely growth rate and requires up to 2 years to blossom. It typically takes 3 to 4 years for your roots to be ready for harvest.

Hops

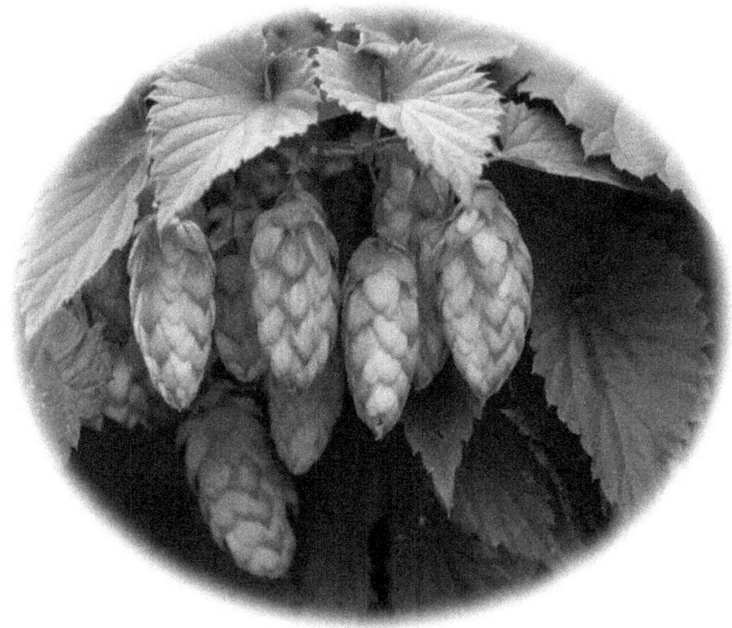

Humulus lupulus

If you've ever felt a pleasantly relaxed state after enjoying a beer with a strong hop flavor, then you're already familiar with the effects of hops. In addition to its calming effects, this herb is known for its ability to reduce nervous tension and anxiety, support digestion, and alleviate bladder discomfort. Hops can help alleviate symptoms of menopause, including hot flashes.

Parts Used: Flowers

Precautions: Due to the presence of a powerful plant estrogen called 8-prenylnaringenin, it is not recommended to administer hops to children who have not yet reached puberty, regardless of their gender. Dogs should avoid consuming hops as they can be harmful.

Identifying/Growing: Hops are cultivated on long vines known as bines, which have the remarkable ability to reach lengths exceeding 25 feet. These lush green plants are not commonly found in the wild. They are usually grown by commercial hops growers who use sturdy trellises to support the bines and ensure proper aeration. The medicinal part of hops is the female flower, which has a pale green color and a cone-like shape.

If you have a sunny spot and vertical space for a sturdy trellis capable of supporting at least 25 pounds, then you might have the opportunity to grow hops in your own backyard. It is recommended to grow at least two varieties to ensure cross-pollination, so it's important to plan accordingly.

Plant the rhizomes in spring, once the risk of frost has passed. Make sure to water them regularly and collect the hops once the cones are filled with a rich, golden powder.

Milk thistle

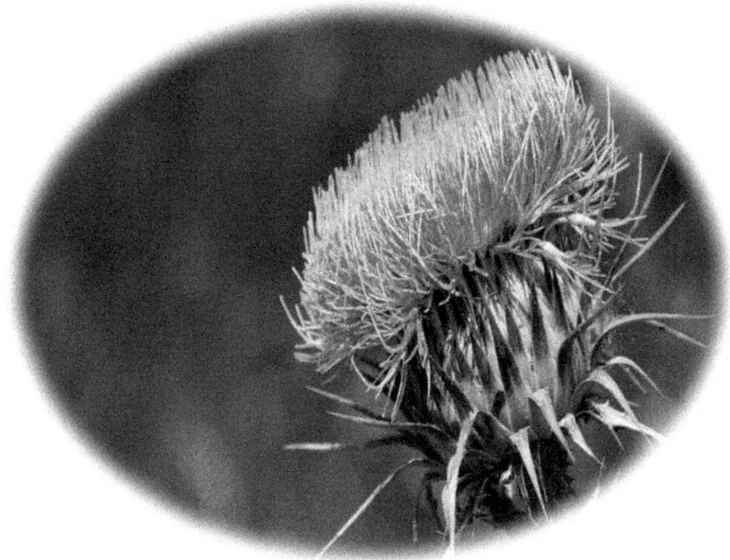

Silybum marianum

Milk thistle's detoxifying properties have made it widely recognized, extending beyond the realm of herbal medicine. This product is enriched with a powerful compound called silymarin, known for its ability to rejuvenate liver cells and shield them from harmful viruses and toxins. If you consume alcohol regularly or engage in the use of strong substances, you may want to consider incorporating milk thistle into your daily routine.

Parts Used: Seeds

Precautions: Overuse can lead to mild diarrhea

Identifying/Growing: Milk thistles can reach an impressive height of 7 feet. With their large, shiny white-veined leaves, these thistle cultivars are easily distinguishable from others. However, their purple flowers bear a striking resemblance.

It's quite simple to cultivate milk thistle in a wide range of climates. For optimal results, it is recommended to sow the seeds either in early spring or late summer. It is important to ensure that the site is adequately watered, allowing the plants to thrive and grow. Make sure to harvest the seed heads once the flowers have faded, before the wind has a chance to carry the seeds away.

Conclusion

There are numerous methods to enhance your understanding of medicinal herbs and their applications for natural healing. For instance, you may be able to locate a local wild crafting class by conducting a brief online search.

If you're looking for a more formal approach to education, you might consider enrolling in a local herbal medicine program. This way, you can gain a wealth of practical information through hands-on learning. If you don't have access to a herbal medicine program or would rather take online courses or conduct your own research, there are alternative options available.

www.ingramcontent.com/pod-product-compliance
Ingram Content Group UK Ltd.
Pitfield, Milton Keynes, MK11 3LW, UK
UKHW062258290726
14090UKWH00017B/769